COMPLEX REGIONAL PAIN SYNDROME (CRPS):

PATIENTS' PERSPECTIVE OF LIVING IN CHRONIC PAIN

Volume II

Alaa Abd-Elsayed M.D., MPH, FASA and Eric M. Phillips

First edition, 2020

Volume II

ISBN: 9798665360508

Other books published by authors:

Alaa Abd-Elsayed

- Chronic Pain: The Patient and Family Journey
- If the Savior is not Safe, How Can He Save?
- Pain: A Review Guide
- Infusion Therapy for Pain, Headache and Related Conditions
- Guide to the inpatient pain consult
- Complex Regional Pain Syndrome (CRPS): Patients' Perspective of Living in Chronic Pain: Volume 1
- Complex Regional Pain Syndrome (CRPS): Patients' Perspective of Living in Chronic Pain: Volume 1-Picture eBook

Eric M. Phillips

- Complex Regional Pain Syndrome (CRPS): Patients' Perspective of Living in Chronic Pain: Volume 1
- Complex Regional Pain Syndrome (CRPS): Patients' Perspective of Living in Chronic Pain: Volume 1-Picture eBook
- Don't Diet: Change Your Eating Habits - Proper Eating for Good Health

Dedication

To my parents, my wife and my two beautiful kids Maro and George.

To all CRPS patients.

Alaa Abd-Elsayed

Dedication

To my loving parents, Janet and my late father Leonard (Lenny) for all their love, and support.

To my beautiful and supportive wife Mercedes, her three children and her grandson.

To my mentor, teacher and greatest friend the late Doctor Hooshang Hooshmand.

To all CRPS patients worldwide.

Eric M. Phillips

TABLE OF CONTENTS

Preface

First, I would like to thank all patients who shared their personal stories with CRPS in this book. We recently published the first volume, which included the stories of several patients who live suffering from CRPS. When we talk about suffering, it is not only pain, but suffering made some patients commit suicide or have an amputation to get rid of the pain.

CRPS is a very serious condition and dealing with it otherwise is not wise. Unfortunately, there is a huge lack of knowledge even among health care providers about the seriousness of this condition and what it can lead to if not managed quickly and aggressively. Early and aggressive management can lead to control and even cure of the pain, but lack of diagnosis and not understanding the urgency of treating this condition can lead to a worsening of pain with associated depression, anxiety, limb atrophy, amputation, and potential suicide.

My friend Eric and I authored volume I and volume II of this book to share the stories of patients suffering from CRPS. Our goal is to increase public awareness of the severity of this condition. What we mean by the public is everyone from employers, spouses, health care providers, and others. It is very important to provide support to CRPS patients to avoid the serious consequences of the condition. Employers should understand the limitations of their employees; "yes, the condition can cause pain to touch," spouses need to support their partners with CRPS, and health care providers should treat it aggressively and quickly. If they have limited experience treating this condition, then they should immediately refer the patient to the experts.

With CRPS, we are racing against time, and providers should start with a non-pharmacological treatment, then medications, and if they fail, then interventions. If one modality is not working, health care providers should move to the next modality without waiting. They should discuss a plan with the patient, with one step after another, and this depends on the success or failure of different modalities.

I hope this book will help increase public awareness about the condition and help CRPS patients to understand the seriousness of this condition and the need to seek help as soon as possible without waiting for too long.

Alaa Abd-Elsayed, MD, MPH, FASA

Preface

I would like to especially thank all the CRPS patients for taking the time to write and share their stories. It is generous of all of you to share your journey of living with this painful disease in this book. Your willingness to share your story will provide great help and support to others who are suffering from CRPS.

I have been working in the CRPS community for over 31-years to help advocate for other CRPS patients. As, being a sufferer of CRPS myself for over 34-years, I understand the struggles and pain that CRPS patients endure. The biggest downfall for most patients is the lack of understanding of CRPS by the medical community and the public.

I have been fortunate to know and work with my friend Doctor Alaa Abd-Elsayed over the years. It has been a great honor for me to work on this second book with Doctor Al and all the patients that were so gracious enough to submit their stories.

We both felt that writing this second book that shared patient's personal stories would help to continue spreading the desperately needed awareness, help educate the public and the medical community that CRPS is a real and serious disease.

I hope this book will be helpful and provide reassurance to other CRPS patients that they are not alone; with their daily battle of dealing with the chronic pain of CRPS. Moreover, I also hope this book will help the medical community worldwide to understand how patients live and cope with this unrelenting painful disease. Remember we all have to work together to help spread awareness in finding a cure for CRPS.

Eric M. Phillips

INTRODUCTION

Alaa Abd-Elsayed, MD, MPH, FASA, and Eric M. Phillips

Complex regional pain syndrome (CRPS), is a poorly understood condition by the medical community. Many patients may suffer long before getting diagnosed or even receive proper treatment.

CRPS is a painful disease that affects the patient physically, mentally, and emotionally. To obtain a complete understanding of this disease, one must read the patient's personal story to get a sense of what can potentially happen to some patients.

As we are all well aware of CRPS is a complex disease to diagnose, treat, and to understand. Treating physicians must take into consideration that each patient is affected differently by CRPS due to the different stages of the disease. The patient and treating physician need to work as a team to create a proper treatment plan that will help the patient control their pain.

CRPS has become a global disease, where there are millions of cases worldwide. CRPS affects patients in the same way. It does not matter if a patient lives in America, Australia, England, France, or anywhere else in this world. Every CRPS patient endures the same chronic pain, have difficulties in receiving proper treatment, and not being believed. Unfortunately, CRPS patients must fight daily to deal with their pain and try to get the recognition that CRPS is a real disease.

We have created this book to help share how patients suffer from the pain of CRPS. Until a doctor, relative, or friend sees the damage that CRPS causes, one cannot comprehend the pain patients deal with daily. These stories you will read in this book range from patients having early stages of the disease to the end-stage of the disease.

The purpose of this book is to help spread awareness about CRPS. Educating the medical community on the topic of CRPS is a high priority. The medical community needs to understand how devastating CRPS is and how it affects the patient physically, mentally, and emotionally.

THE MISCONCEPTIONS OF COMPLEX REGIONAL PAIN SYNDROME (CRPS)

Eric M. Phillips

International RSD Foundation

www.rsdinfo.com

Abstract: *Complex regional pain syndrome (CRPS), is a poorly misunderstood disease. There are many misconceptions about how CRPS affects patients on many levels, from diagnosis of the disease to selecting a proper treatment plan for the patient.*

It is unfortunate, that patients have to live life in constant chronic pain from CRPS and have to endure seeing physicians who have a poor understanding of the disease. There is a small majority of physicians who have an understanding of CRPS.

Keywords: *Complex regional pain syndrome (CRPS), misconceptions of CRPS, and spread of CRPS.*

Introduction

For decades, physicians have recognized complex regional pain syndrome (CRPS), as a rare disease. CRPS is no longer considered a rare disease. There is a higher prevalence of reported cases of the disease, which affects millions of people worldwide. The lack of understanding of the disease by the medical community can cause serious issues for the patient.

Hence, these facts can lead to misdiagnosis, wrong treatment, or no treatment at all. These delays in receiving proper help can lead to many years of suffering for the patient.

6

There are many misconceptions associated with CRPS that can cause issues for many patients. This article will discuss these misconceptions that physicians apply to the diagnosis, symptoms, and treatment of CRPS.

Misconceptions of CRPS

Some physicians who treat CRPS patients have many misconceptions about the aspects of the disease, i.e., the development of CRPS, signs, and symptoms of the disease, duration of CRPS, and spread of the disease.

Over the past 31-years of working in the CRPS community and speaking with thousands of CRPS patients each year, I have heard first-hand all of the misconceptions of CRPS that physicians tell their patients.

Below is a list of some important misconceptions that some physicians believe are true in the management or (mismanagement) of CRPS.

- **The CRPS does not spread misconception**: One of the top misconceptions of CRPS is that most physicians do not believe that CRPS can spread. Research work by Doctors Hooshmand, Schwartzman, Veldman, Merskey and others, have all recognized that CRPS can spread to other parts of the body, including the internal organs (1-13). This is an important fact that the disease can spread in some cases. When physicians discount the fact the CRPS can spread, it causes the patient to have more pain, and it can potentially cause a delay in receiving proper treatment which can provide adequate pain relief and prevent further spread of the disease. Please read more under the topic of the spread of CRPS.
- **You have a "mild case of CRPS" misconception:** Some patients are informed that they have a "mild case of CRPS." There is no such thing as a mild case of CRPS. Physicians should take all cases of

CRPS seriously. A mild case of CRPS today will become a serve case of CRPS tomorrow if not treated promptly and properly. This misconception can cause a lot of harm to a patient when they are newly diagnosed.

- **Your CRPS will burn-out misconception:** Some physicians have a misconception that CRPS is will burn-out in 12-18 months. This is another misconception that gives patients false hope. In very rare cases, some patient's symptoms may go into remission. But, for the majority of CRPS patients, they live years in chronic pain.

- **The signs and symptoms of CRPS misconception:** Some physicians treating CRPS feel that a patient has to have every sign and symptom on the list to be diagnosed with CRPS. This is another false and misleading misconception of CRPS. As most patients and physicians know the symptoms of CRPS can come and go at any given time. The main symptoms that should be taken into consideration to give a valid and proper diagnosis are the following symptoms. Burning pain in the extremity caused by a minor trauma or surgery, ice-cold pain in the extremity caused by minor trauma or surgery, discoloration of the skin, swelling (edema) of the extremity, and hypersensitivity of the skin (allodynia). If any of these symptoms are present, then one must give the diagnosis of CRPS. As mentioned before the patient does not have to have all these symptoms at the same time. The two most important and vital symptoms of this disease are the burning pain or the ice-cold pain in the affected extremity. In the beginning stages of CRPS, most symptoms are not all present at the same time. This misconception can cause the patient to be misdiagnosed for many years and cause irreversible damage from not being properly diagnosed and treated.

- **The CRPS stages misconception:** Some physicians have a misconception about the staging of CRPS. They feel that there are only three stages of the disease and they don't understand that stages can vary in their duration. According to my mentor, the late Doctor Hooshmand, there are four stages associated with CRPS. Stage I: sympathetic dysfunction, Stage II: dystrophy, Stage III: atrophy, and Stage IV: failure of the immune system (1). Please read more under the topic of stages of CRPS.

- **The "drug seeker" misconception:** Some physicians believe CRPS patients are simply "drug seekers." This is another false and misleading misconception that harms the patient. CRPS patients are not drug seekers, they are only seeking pain relief. In most cases, the strongest pain medications will not help relieve the patient's pain. Patients suffering from CRPS should be treated with strong analgesics, which are not addicting. Strong non-addicting pain medications such as Buprenorphine, Stadol, and Ultram, which are helpful and a safer alternative in the treatment of CRPS (14).

Antidepressants are the analgesic of choice for treatment of persistent and long-standing pain for any cause. The use of antidepressants such as desipramine or trazodone is quite helpful because they provide analgesia (relief of pain) which can be very beneficial in helping the pain and symptoms of CRPS (14).

Nonsteroidal anti-inflammatory medications such as Mobic (meloxicam), Voltaren (diclofenac) (gel or tablet), Celebrex (celecoxib), and Anaprox (naproxen) are quite helpful in treating the neuro-inflammation of CRPS (14).

The use of muscle relaxants is another important part of the treatment plan for CRPS patients who suffer from muscle spasms. The ideal muscle relaxant in the treatment of CRPS is Lioresal (baclofen) which helps relax the muscles as well as taking away the flexion spasms (14).

Adding Anticonvulsants to the game plan, especially Tegretol (carbamazepine) (non-generic), Depakene (valproic acid), Gabapentin and Klonopin (non-generic), are quite effective in treating CRPS (14-19).

Physicians who have the misconception that CRPS patients are just drug seekers, need to learn to think outside of the box. They need to understand that there are other safer medication alternatives that they can offer patients for treatment, so they can obtain safe and quality pain relief.

- **The "CRPS is all in your head" misconception:** One of the biggest and most frustrating misconceptions is when the physician mentions to the patient that "CRPS is all in their head." This is a false misconception. Psychological factors do not cause CRPS. Having CRPS may create some psychological factors such as depression and other emotional distress in some patients. It would not be normal if any patient suffering from CRPS, cancer, or any other debilitating condition not be depressed or have some emotional reaction to their disease.

Children suffering from CRPS receive a tremendous amount of disbelief in their symptoms and pain. They are most often labeled as being too emotional, depressed, school phobic, upset about their family life if they have parents who are going through a divorce, or if they suffer from another illness or conditions. Their CRPS is blamed on psychological factors, not on the initial injury that caused their CRPS.

In Doctor Hooshmand's review of 824 CRPS patients, one or more of the limbic system dysfunctions were present in every case except three. These consisted of insomnia (92%), irritability, agitation, anxiety (78%), (depression (73%), poor memory and concentration (48%), poor judgment (36%), and panic attacks (32%) (20). Understanding the nature of the emotional components of CRPS spares the patient from misdiagnosis and improper treatment (2,20).

According to De Good et al., reported patients suffering from CRPS, when compared to patients suffering from back pain and headaches, had the highest level of pain intensity but demonstrated relatively less emotional distress (20,21).

However, because of the nihilistic approach of the neurologists regarding any form of chronic disease, causing neuropsychological dysfunction, the CRPS patients are frequently called neurotic, and histrionic (20).

There is no doubt that the CRPS affects the limbic system invariably causes psychological disturbances including tendencies for being neurotic, histrionic, exaggeration, poor judgment, poor memory, poor concentration, and depression. Yet the CRPS patient is expected to be stoic, and to be able to sleep through the constant protopathic and allodynic pain. Otherwise, the patient is considered to have a "psychiatric disturbance (20)."

In practically, every patient suffering from CRPS demonstrates some degree of the limbic system disturbance. These patients are expected to be depressed in more than three-quarters of the cases, are anxious in practically every one of the cases, and suffer from insomnia, agitation, irritability and poor judgment in practically every one of the cases. These manifestations are one of the four criteria for the diagnosis of CRPS. There is no way the limbic system can be left intact in the face of CRPS. (20).

The fact remains that regardless of whatever the nihilist wants to call it, be it, RSD, CRPS, Mimocausalgia, or any other name, the CRPS based on the above mentioned four principles have a stereotyped clinical picture that cannot be mistaken for any other disease. This is a diagnosis made on the so-called "Four Duck Principle (Table I)." The well-known Four Duck Principle describes "if it waddles like a duck, quacks like a duck, looks like a duck, and is called a duck, then it must be a duck."

With proper understanding, the nature of the emotional components of CRPS spares the patient from years of misdiagnosis and improper treatment (20).

Table I. The Four Duck Principle
Principle 1: Afferent: Allodynia, hyperpathia.
Principle 2: Efferent: Muscle spasm, cold extremities, paresis, tremors.
Principle 3: Inflammation: Edema, ulcers, skin rash, MRSA.
Principle 4: Limbic System: Dysfunction, poor memory, poor judgment, insomnia, and depression.

- **The "you look too good to have CRPS" misconception:** This misconception is when a physician tells the patient that they look too good, too pretty or too healthy to have CRPS. Since there is a higher percentage of women who have CRPS, why would their appearance of being a pretty woman or, looking too healthy to have CRPS have any bearing on their level of pain? Just because a patient looks pretty or looks healthy should not discount their symptoms or pain. I am sure that there are many pretty and healthy-looking cancer patients out there. Does their appearance as a cancer patient discount their pain and suffering? I remember a patient that we saw at Doctor Hooshmand's clinic telling us about her experience with her pain doctor. He made a comment to her that she looked too pretty to have CRPS. She said that she was highly insulted by his comments. I told this patient that she should have said to this doctor, that he looked too dumb and acted too ignorant to be a doctor.

- **The misconceptions of treatment:** Most physicians have a misconception that patients should only have three to six stellate ganglion nerve blocks or lower lumbar sympathetic nerve blocks. Then, they offer the patient either a spinal cord stimulator (SCS), sympathectomy (surgical, chemical or radio-frequency), or an infusion pump. Other alternative treatments that should be considered before any surgical intervention should take place. Many other types of nerve blocks that can be beneficial in the treatment of CRPS.

Doctor Hooshmand, et al, found the use of epidural nerve blocks (ENB) is the last resort type of nerve block for patients suffering from late-stage chronic CRPS. He and his team, have found that CRPS patients gain the most benefit from treatment with ENB compared to treatment with standard SGB.

Paravertebral nerve blocks (PNB) are another helpful and safe form of nerve blocks in the treatment of CRPS. The PNB is applied in the paravertebral muscles (muscles on each side of the midline of the vertebrae in the back or neck). The injection is done around the sensory nerves that are transmitting the pain to the spinal cord.

This is in contrast to the other types of blocks lasting more than nine weeks (Table II) (22).

- The epidural blocks containing Depo-Medrol® were successful in 89% of patients.

- The regional Bier blocks showed an average success rate of 32%.

- The brachial plexus blocks showed a 63% success in regards to analgesia and hyperthermia.

Treatment for late stages of CRPS should consist of using ENB, PNB, and trigger point injection as safer alternatives to using repetitive SGB in the management of CRPS.

Table II. Comparison of Nerve Blocks (22).	
Type of Nerve Block	**Duration of Pain Relief**
Sympathetic Ganglion Block	11 ± 2 days
Epidural Steroid Block	9 ± 5 weeks
Regional Bier Block	2 ± 1 weeks
Brachial Plexus Block	8 ± 2 weeks

- **The discrimination misconception:** CRPS does not discriminate. It does not matter what, race, color, religion, or creed a patient is. Nor does it matter what profession the patient works in. In 2000, I attended a medical conference on CRPS with my mentor Doctor Hooshmand. I was amazed when a doctor attending the conference asked the question of why "professionals" (doctors, or lawyers) don't develop CRPS? My jaw almost hit the floor when I heard that question. This doctor has the misconception that only non-professionals develop CRPS. This is another false and misleading misconception. In my 31-years of working in the CRPS community, I have talked with many people who are doctors, lawyers, nurses, therapists, church ministers, pastors, and other professionals who have all developed CRPS. It does not matter what your profession is. The bottom line is CRPS does not discriminate. Sadly, some physicians still believe the misconception that CRPS only happens to non-professionals.

- **The "doctor shopping" misconception:** Some physicians have the misconception that patients are just "doctor shopping" to get medication. This is another false and misleading misconception. A majority of physicians misdiagnosed CRPS patients with other conditions. This is the reason that many patients have to see multiple doctors before they find the right doctor for proper diagnosis of CRPS. In other cases, patients have to find new doctors because their treating pain doctor leaves the practice or moves out of state. The other reason why patients search for other doctors is that it's just not a good fit between the doctor and patient. Another reason could be that the treatments are no longer working for the patient or that the doctor has run out of options to help treat the patient. This causes the patient to start the process over again to find a new doctor to search for more answers and obtain help and pain relief. This is another misconception that is harmful to the patient's overall health. One must remember CRPS patients are only seeking the right answers and to find the proper help to relieve their pain.

- **The misconception that CRPS does not cause disturbance of the immune system:** A majority of physicians have the misconception that CRPS does not cause disturbance of the immune system. This is another false misconception. In many CRPS cases, patients do develop a compromised immune system due to their CRPS. This is a severe complication of the disease that affects many patients. Physicians need to understand that this is a real important complication of CRPS and it should be taken seriously and treated promptly.

Doctor Hooshmand and I co-authored an article in which, we reported that the sympathetic system regulates the immune system. The sympathetic system is responsible for the control of body temperature, control of vital signs and control of the immune system. Any kind of stress that stimulates the sympathetic system also stimulates the immune system (3).

In the first two years after the development of CRPS, the immune system is upregulated with high T cell lymphocytes causing low-grade fever, neurodermatitis, trophic ulcers, spontaneous bruising, edema, clinical pictures of compression (entrapment), and neuropathies such as so-called carpal tunnel syndrome and thoracic ulcer syndrome, which can easily be corrected with conservative treatment rather than surgical treatment (3).

After two years, as the CRPS becomes chronic and the healing power (plasticity) of the nervous system and the immune system becomes disturbed. The patient develops a hypoactive, down-regulated immune system with the development of permanent elevation of killer T cell lymphocytes, suppression of helper T cell lymphocytes, and development of persistent skin pathology, such as persistent edema involving the paraspinal and upper and lower extremities. The patient also develops persistent pruritus and neurodermatitis, persistent trophic ulcers, spontaneous bruising, permanent dystrophic changes regarding skin healing, and abnormal hair and nail growth (3).

CRPS is due to dysfunction of the sympathetic nervous system. The sympathetic nerves function dynamically at times being hyperactive and at other times being hypoactive. This is regarding the control of circulation and control of the immune system. From day to day the sympathetic control of circulation may fluctuate. This is usually in the form of neurovascular instability, meaning one day the hand or foot is bluish red, and the next day it is so white it looks like it is dead. The immune system control may undergo up-regulation or down-regulation: one day the patient is feverish, and the next day the patient is "ice-cold" (3).

According to Doctor Hooshmand's research, it examines that in the first few months of abnormal sympathetic function (acute CRPS during the first six months) the sympathetic and parasympathetic systems show significant plasticity and can adjust their activities to preserve the immune system. However, after two to three years, (chronic CRPS) this power of plasticity and ability to fluctuate the balance of the immune system disappears. As a result, the immune function is thrown off balance with resultant development of frequent infections, and in the long run, the development of a tendency for cancer. Certain treatments influence the plasticity and the balance of the two systems positively or negatively (23).

Doctor Hooshmand reported that the following are the treatments that deteriorate the immune function (23).

- Unnecessary surgery. This is especially true in the case of CRPS involving the hand or foot, causing inflammation and swelling at the wrist or ankle mimicking the clinical picture of carpal tunnel or tarsal tunnel syndrome. Surgery at the wrist or ankle in such patients aggravates the condition tremendously and weakens the immune system. Sticking needles and giving injections in the swollen areas of carpal tunnel or tarsal tunnel also accelerates the deterioration of the immune system and should be avoided.

- Intake of drugs such as alcohol, addicting narcotics, and addicting BZs.

- Continuous distress due to the legal entanglements related to the trauma that initially caused CRPS.

- Inactivity and lack of exercise.

- Certain, so-called foods such as hot dogs. It has been shown that children who eat more than four hot dogs a week have five times higher incidence of suffering from a cancerous brain tumor than the children who do not eat hot dogs.

- The use of ice on the extremity accelerates the constriction of the blood vessels and aggravates the CRPS hastening the development of the disturbance of the immune system.

Any measure taken in the opposite direction will prevent deterioration of the function of the immune system.

Doctor Hooshmand's, recommendation for treatments is in the form of nerve blocks, antidepressants that provide natural REM sleep (such as Trazodone), and physiotherapy along with the application of moist heat to prevent the disturbance of the immune system (23).

Once the patient develops the picture of disturbance of the immune system, treatment with medications such as I.V. Immunoglobulin (IVIG) or Adrenocorticotropic hormone (ACTH) may be helpful. Even though corticosteroids such as Prednisone or Decadron slow down the abnormal function of the immune system, they tend to result in atrophy of the adrenal glands. The atrophy of the adrenal glands aggravates the function of the immune system (23).

ACTH in judicious doses does not cause atrophy of the adrenal glands and have beneficial effects both on the immune system and on reducing the swelling of the soft tissues secondary to CRPS. One of the complications of CRPS, especially after the immune system is disturbed, is the development of frequent attacks of neurodermatitis, skin rash, and breakdown of the skin (23).

Medications such as Zonalon (topical Doxepin) and topical TAC (tetracaine, adrenaline, cocaine) help counteract the skin breakdown in such patients. Another similar topical lotion called LAT (Lidocaine-adrenaline-tetracaine) is similarly effective. The use of Epsom salt (magnesium sulfate) and warm water can help reduce swelling. In some advanced acute stages of the disease, Capsaicin may be helpful. Using a Clonidine Patch at any stage of CRPS is an effective form of treatment, not only for the skin dysfunction but, also as a sympathetic nerve block agent (23).

- **The misconception that surgery is safe for CRPS patients:** Many physicians have the misconception that surgery is safe for CRPS patients. This is another false and misleading misconception that will cause the patient more harm.
  Surgery can cause more harm and spread of the disease. Patients need to avoid any unnecessary surgery due to the high risk that their CRPS will spread and cause more pain.

The commonest forms of surgical procedures that cause permanent damage and permanent intractability of CRPS are (24):

- Carpal tunnel surgery.
- Tarsal tunnel surgery.

- Rotator cuff surgery.
- Ulnar nerve decompression.
- Surgical exploration of the knee, neuroma, or ankle.
- Thoracic outlet syndrome surgery.
- Removal of a bulging disc or herniated discs in the distribution of spasm and pain secondary to CRPS.

Over the years, we have seen the spread of the disease in patients who have undergone surgical sympathectomy (be it surgical, chemical, or radiofrequency). Any type of sympathectomy is useless for advanced cases of CRPS. It will cause a rapid spread of CRPS to other parts of the body and cause more pain for the patient.

Surgery for the infusion pump or the spinal cord stimulator (SCS) also causes the spread of the disease. These implants are apt to fail and cause more pain for the patient.

In Doctor Hooshmand's review article of 824 CRPS cases, he states there are times that surgery is unavoidable (20). Examples: tear of a ligament or cartilage in the knee joint that would preclude weight-bearing. In such patients, epidural nerve block with a combination of Bupivacaine and 20 to 30 mg Prednisolone before, during, and after surgery (with the help of an epidural catheter) helps reduce the side effects of surgical trauma. Another example is an extensor deformity of a finger, causing a useless hand, which in turn aggravates CRPS (20).

Patients and physicians must have an open line of communication when the topic of having unnecessary surgery is discussed. Having any type of surgery can be a high risk for any CRPS patient.

It is better to have all the facts in place before having any surgery that could potentially spread the CRPS. Avoiding surgery can help spare the patient from the unwanted spread of the disease.

- **The misconception that CRPS cannot cause other complications:** Some physicians have the misconception that CRPS cannot cause other complications. This is another false misconception. Over the last few decades, we have seen and have reported many patients developing other complications that are connected with CRPS. These complications are seen in patients who have had CRPS for many years to decades. Physicians need to understand that these other complications associated with CRPS are real. These complications should be treated and addressed, not ignored. The CRPS patient suffers enough from the daily pain of the disease. They do not need to suffer from other complications.

As Doctor Hooshmand and I have reported in the article Various Complications of CRPS, we found most patients suffer from the standard signs and symptoms of CRPS (3). Over time a majority of patients that have suffered for many years to decades do develop various complications of the disease. Over the years we have recognized a large array of various complications associated with CRPS which often go untreated. Many of these complications are not well recognized by the medical community. However, CRPS continues to be a very complex disease to understand and to treat. These various complications can impede the proper treatment for the spread of the disease and the underlying issues that arise from these complications (3).

It is well known that during the long duration of the disease when patients reach stage IV, they start to develop various complications such as disturbance of the immune system (neurogenic inflammation), limbic system, cardiac system, the endocrine system, and the respiratory system. These are just a few of the various complications of CRPS (3).

Table III describes the other complications that are associated with CRPS. Few physicians recognized these complications (Table III) (1,2,3,25,26).

Table III. Various Complications of CRPS (3)	
Agitation	Internal Organ Involvement
Cardiac Disturbance	Interstitial Cystitis
Depression	Intractable Hypertension
Disturbance of the Immune System	Irritability
Disturbance of Judgment	Keratitis Sicca (Dry Eyes)
Dysphagia	Limbic System Dysfunction
Endocrine System Dysfunction	Low Cortisol Levels
Fatigue	Movement Disorders
Gardner Diamond Syndrome (Spontaneous Bruising)	Respiratory System Complications
Gastrointestinal Complications	Skin Lesions, Rashes, and Ulcers
GERDS	Spread of CRPS
Headaches (Migraine)	Tinnitus
Hearing Complications	Urological Complications
Hypothyroidism	Visual Disturbance
Insomnia	Vulvodynia

Stages of CRPS

According to Doctor Hooshmand, et al, CRPS has been divided into four different stages (2,3).

Depending on the nature of the injury, the stages vary in their duration. In Doctor Hooshmand's review of 824 CRPS patients, 17 patients suffering from Venipuncture CRPS showed, deterioration from stage I to stage III was measured in a few weeks up to less than nine months. This is in contrast with CRPS in children in which stages would stagnate, reverse or improve slowly (2,3).

Stage I: is a sympathetic dysfunction with the typical thermatomal distribution of the pain. The pain may spread in a mirror fashion to the contralateral extremity or adjacent regions on the same side of the body (5). In stage one; the pain is usually SMP in nature.

The complex regional pain and inflammation spread to other extremities in approximately one-third of CRPS patients (2,3,27-29).

In stage II: the dysfunction changes to dystrophy manifested by edema, hyperhidrosis, neurovascular instability with fluctuation of livedo reticularis and cyanosis - causing the change of temperature and color of the skin in a matter of minutes. The dystrophic changes also include bouts of hair loss, ridging, dystrophic, brittle and discolored nails, skin rash, subcutaneous bleeding, neurodermatitis, and ulcerative lesions.

At stage II or III: it is not at all uncommon for CRPS to spread to other extremities (2,3,30,31). At times, it may become generalized. The generalized CRPS is an infrequent late-stage complication (2,3,5). It is accompanied by sympathetic dysfunction in all four extremities as well as attacks of headache, vertigo, poor memory, and poor concentration.

The spread through paravertebral and midline sympathetic nerves may be vertical, horizontal, or both (2,3,5,31-33).

Stage IV identifies the final stage of CRPS manifested by (1-3):

- Failure of the immune system, reduction of helper T-cell lymphocytes and elevation of killer T-cell lymphocytes.

- Intractable hypertension changes to orthostatic hypotension (2,3,34).

- Intractable generalized edema involving the abdomen, pelvis, lungs, and extremities.

- Ulcerative skin lesions which may respond to treatment with I.V. Mannitol, I.V. Immunoglobulin, and ACTH treatments. Calcium channel blockers such as Nifedipine may be effective in the treatment (2,3,35).

- High risks of cancer and suicide are increased.

- Multiple surgical procedures seem to be precipitating factors for the development of stage IV. Stage IV is almost the flip side of earlier stages and points to exhaustion of autonomic and immune systems.

- With the passage of time and types of treatment, CRPS goes through stages with variable timetables and sympathetic responses (2,3,35) (Table IV).

Table IV. The average duration of development from stage I to stage III (3).	
Types of CRPS	**Duration**
VP CRPS II (17 Patients)	4 ½ months
CRPS treated with amputation	10 months
CRPS after carpal tunnel surgery	14 months
CRPS in electrical injury	25 months
CRPS treated with no surgery	29 months

Spread of CRPS

For decades there has been a lot of scrutiny by the medical community regarding the spread of CRPS. There have been many published articles reporting that it is not uncommon for CRPS to spread. A majority of patients' have experienced spread into other parts of their bodies over time. The spread of CRPS can occur during stages II, III and IV of the disease (2,3,5,30,31).

According to Kozin et al., CRPS can spread vertically or horizontally in both upper or both lower extremities (31,35). Also, undergoing any surgical procedure can promote the potential spread of CRPS (30,36). Maleki et al. published a retrospective analysis of 27 CRPS patients. In this study, all 27 patients had experienced a spread of their pain (36-38). Doctor Hooshmand, reported the chain of sympathetic ganglia from the base of the skull to sacral regions on the right and left sides, typically spread the pathologic impulse to other extremities (1). The observed phenomenon of referred pain of CRPS can sometimes be mistaken for the spread of the disease. These are two separate issues that patients go through.

Usual factors that can facilitate the spread of CRPS are surgical procedures, the application of ice, and the stress of too much activity, or inactivity (2). In Doctor Hooshmand's review of 824 CRPS patients, the number one aggravator was cryosurgery, followed by surface cryotherapy applied for over two months, showed the spread of the disease (11,36). The surface cryotherapy less than two months did not show the tendency for the spread of CRPS (2,11,36).

CRPS can involve internal organs. The attacks of swelling of the internal organs complicated by intermittent constriction of the blood vessels to different organs can cause chest pain, attacks of sharp central pain (stabbing severe pain in the chest or abdomen), and changes in the voice (suddenly developing a temporary "chipmunk" type of voice change). The use of anticonvulsants such as Tegretol or Neurontin can relieve the sharp, stabbing central pain (36).

We have seen patients with internal organ complications. These complications can develop by the traumatic effect of a sympathetic nerve block. This complication is caused by accidental trauma to the kidney with resultant hematuria (blood in urine) and aggravation of hypertension (36).

Physicians who treat CRPS patients should not overlook or dismiss the fact CRPS can spread to other parts of the body or the internal organs (36). Avoiding any unnecessary surgeries, and the application of ice helps prevent the spread of CRPS. (2,11). If the symptoms of spread are present, the physician should provide the proper treatment with nerve blocks, strong non-addicting pain medications, antidepressants, and nonsteroidal anti-inflammatory medications to help treat the new symptoms caused by the spread of the disease.

Conclusion

CRPS is a complex disease to diagnose, treat, and manage. The many misconceptions that some physicians apply to CRPS can cause the patient many years of disbelief of their symptoms and pain, and lack of proper treatment.

These important misconceptions of CRPS discussed in this chapter can cause the patient more harm, more pain, more stress, and causes mistrust in the treating physician and the medical community.

To help prevent these misconceptions of CRPS in the future, we need to educate the medical community. There have been many published medical articles and books on the topic of CRPS that proves the disease can spread, cause various complications and many other side-effects of the disease.

I have always said CRPS is not "rocket science." These misconceptions of CRPS create mismanagement of the disease, which causes the patient more pain, and stress. Patients must find a physician who understands CRPS. Both the patient and physician need to work as a team to achieve the main goal for the patient to be pain-free and have a better quality of life.

I would like to share a great quote that was written by my mentor and best friend, the late Doctor Hooshang Hooshmand.

To all CRPS Patients: "Remember, CRPS is not all in your head." It is all over your body. It starts from one extremity or one part of the body, and if not properly treated, it spreads to the other parts of the body. Do not let anybody convince you to be treated exclusively by a psychiatrist or to learn to live with your pain.

Just remember you are not crazy. The pain of CRPS is enough to drive anybody out of their mind, but what I admire is the fact that CRPS patients still keep their sanity.   H. Hooshmand, M. D.

References

1. Hooshmand H. Chronic Pain: Reflex Sympathetic Dystrophy: Prevention and Management. CRC Press, Boca Raton FL. 1993.

2.Hooshmand H, Hashmi H. Complex regional pain syndrome (CRPS, RSDS) diagnosis and therapy. A review of 824 patients. Pain Digest 1999; 9:1-24. http://www.rsdrx.com/CRPS_824_Patients_Article.pdf

3.Hooshmand H, Phillips EM. Various Complications of Complex Regional Pain Syndrome (CRPS). Neurological Associates Pain Management Center, Vero Beach, Florida. www.rsdinfo.com and www.rsdrx.com Feb 16, 2016.

4. Schwartzman RJ. Systemic complications of complex regional pain syndrome. Neuroscience & Medicine 2012, 3, 225-242. http://www.scirp.org/journal/PaperInformation.aspx?paperID=22695

5. Veldman PH, Goris R.J. Multiple reflex sympathetic dystrophy. Which patients are at risk for developing a recurrence of reflex sympathetic dystrophy in the same or another limb? Pain 1996 Mar; 64(3):463-466. http://journals.lww.com/pain/Abstract/1996/03000/Multiple_reflex_sym pathetic_dystrophy__Which.8.aspx

6. Merskey H, Bogduk N. Classification of Chronic Pain Descriptions of Chronic Pain Syndromes and Definitions of Pain Terms. Task Force on Taxonomy of the International Association for the Study of Pain. Merskey, H. editor. IASP Press. Seattle 1994. http://www.iasp-

pain.org/files/Content/ContentFolders/Publications2/FreeBooks/Classific
ation-ofChronic-Pain.pdf

7. Dielissen PW, Claassen AT, Veldman PH, et al. Amputation for reflex
sympathetic dystrophy. J Bone Joint Surg 1995 ; 77 :270-3.
http://www.ncbi.nlm.nih.gov/pubmed/7706345

8. Veldman PH, Goris RJ. Surgery on extremities with reflex sympathetic
dystrophy. Unfallchirurg 1995; 98:45-48.
http://www.ncbi.nlm.nih.gov/pubmed/7886464

9. Schwartzman RJ, McLellan TL. Reflex sympathetic dystrophy. A review.
Arch Neurol 1987; 44: 555- 561.
http://archneur.jamanetwork.com/article.aspx?articleid=586446

10. Livingston WK. Pain mechanisms: A physiological interpretation of
causalgia and its related states. In London, MacMillan 1944.

11. Hooshmand, H, Hashmi, M, Phillips, EM. Cryotherapy can cause
permanent nerve damage: A case report. AJPM 2004; 14: 2: 63-70.
http://www.rsdinfo.com/Cryotherapy_Article.pdf

12. Hooshmand H, Phillips EM. Complex regional pain syndrome (CRPS)-
Reflex sympathetic dystrophy (RSD) diagnosis and management protocol.
2009. 1-14. www.rsdrx.com and www.rsdinfo.com

13. Veldman PH, Reynen HM, Arntz IE, et al. Signs and symptoms of reflex
sympathetic dystrophy: prospective study of 829 patients. Lancet 1993;
342:1012-1016. http://www.ncbi.nlm.nih.gov/pubmed/8105263

14. Hooshmand H, (Retired) and Phillips EM. Medication in the
management of complex regional pain syndrome (CRPS). Jun 8, 2017.
www.rsdrx.com and www.rsdinfo.com

15. McQuay H, Carroll D, Jada AR, et al. Anticonvulsant drugs for management of pain: a systemic review. BMJ 1995; 311:1047-1052
http://www.bmj.com/content/311/7012/1047.long 3

16. Mellick GA, Mellick LB. Reflex sympathetic dystrophy treated with gabapentin. Arch Phys Med Rehabil 1997; 78:98-105
http://www.archives-pmr.org/article/S0003-9993(97)90020-4/pdf

17. Swerdlow M, Cundill JG. Anticonvulsant drugs used in the treatment of lancinating pain. A comparison. Anaesthesia 1981; 36:1129-1132
https://www.ncbi.nlm.nih.gov/pubmed/6798892 13

18. Reddy S, Patt RB. The benzodiazepines as adjuvant analgesics. J Pain Symptom Manage 1994; 9:510-514
http://www.sciencedirect.com/science/article/pii/0885392494901120

19. Hooshmand H. Intractable seizures. Treatment with a new benzodiazepine anticonvulsant. Arch Neurol 1972; 27:205-208
http://jamanetwork.com/journals/jamaneurology/articleabstract/571613

20. Hooshmand H, Phillips EM. Psychological aspects of reflex sympathetic dystrophy (RSD)-complex regional pain syndrome (CRPS). Source : www.rsdrx.com and www.rsdinfo.com

21. De Good DE, Cundiff GW, Adams LE, et al. A psychosocial and behavioral comparison of reflex sympathetic dystrophy, low back pain, and headache patients. Pain 1993; 54: 317-22.

22. Hooshmand, H, Hashmi, M, and Phillips, E.M. Nerve Blocks for Neuropathic Pain. Abstracts of the 10th World Congress on Pain. San Diego, California, August 19, 2002. International Association for the Study of Pain (IASP Press) Page 208, Number 638- P272.
https://www.rsdinfo.com/RSD-Articles/Nerve_Block_Abstract.pdf

23. Hooshmand H. RSD Puzzle #35: My RSD is four years old. I have recently started having frequent infections and my doctor tells me that my immune system is not functioning properly. Can RSD cause this problem? Source: www.rsdrx.com 1997.

24. Hooshmand H and Phillips EM. The management of complex regional pain syndrome (CRPS). Neurological Associates Pain Management Center, Vero Beach, Florida. www.rsdinfo.com and www.rsdrx.com Jan 24, 2010.

25. Hooshmand H, Phillips, EM. Repetitive strain injury (RSI) diagnosis and treatment. 2009; 1-12. www.rsdrx.com and www.rsdinfo.com

26. Schwartzman RJ, Erwin KL, et al. "The natural history of complex regional pain syndrome," The Clinical Journal of Pain 2009, Vol. 25, No. 4, 273-280. http://www.ncbi.nlm.nih.gov/pubmed/19590474

27. Chelimsky T, Low PA, Naessens JM, et al. Value of autonomic testing in reflex sympathetic dystrophy. Mayo Clinic Proceedings 1995; 70:1029-1040. https://www.mayoclinicproceedings.org/article/S0025-6196(11)64438-8/abstract

28. Fredriksen TA, Hovdal H, Sjaastad O. "Cervicogenic headache": clinical manifestation. Cephalalgia 1987; 7:147-160. http://cep.sagepub.com/content/7/2/147.abstract

29. Moskowitz MA. The neurobiology of vascular head pain. Ann Neurol 1984 ; 16 :157-168. http://www.ncbi.nlm.nih.gov/pubmed/6206779

30. Radt P. Bilateral reflex neurovascular dystrophy following a neurosurgical procedure. Clinical picture and therapeutic problems of the syndrome. Confin Neurol 1968; 30:341- 348. https://www.karger.com/Article/Pdf/103547

31. Kozin F, McCarty DJ, Sims J, et al. The reflex sympathetic dystrophy syndrome. I. Clinical and histologic studies: Evidence of bilaterality, response to corticosteroids and articular involvement. Am J Med 1976; 60:321- 331.
http://www.ncbi.nlm.nih.gov/pubmed/56891?dopt=Abstract

32. Duncan KH, Lewis RC, Racz G, et al. Treatment of upper extremity reflex sympathetic dystrophy with joint stiffness using sympathetic bier blocks and manipulation. Orthopedics 1988 ; 11 :883-886.
http://www.ncbi.nlm.nih.gov/pubmed/3387335

33. Cayla J, Rondier J. Algodystrophies reflexes des membres inferieurs d'origine vertebroipelvienne (a propos de 23 cas). Sem Hop 1974; 50:275-286. http://www.ncbi.nlm.nih.gov/pubmed/4368242

34. Polinsky RJ. Shy-Drager syndrome. In: Jankovic J, Tolosa E, eds. Parkinson's disease and movement disorders. 2nd ed. Baltimore: Williams and Wilkins. 1993, pp 191-204.

35. Webster CF, Schwartzman RJ, Jacoby RA, et al. Reflex sympathetic dystrophy. Occurrence of inflammatory skin lesions in patients with stages II and III disease. Arch Dermatol 1991;127: 1541-1544.
http://www.ncbi.nlm.nih.gov/pubmed/8425967

36. Hooshmand H, Phillips, EM. Spread of complex regional pain syndrome (CRPS). 2009; 1-11. www.rsdrx.com and www.rsdinfo.com

37. Schwartzman RJ. Reflex sympathetic dystrophy. Handbook of Clinical Neurology. Spinal Cord Trauma, H.L. Frankel, editor. Elsevier Science Publisher B.V. 1992; 17: 121-136.

38. Maleki J, LeBel AA, Bennett GJ, Schwartzman RJ. Patterns of Spread of complex regional pain syndrome, type I (reflex sympathetic dystrophy). Pain 2000; 88: 259-266.
https://journals.lww.com/pain/Abstract/2000/12010/Patterns_of_spread_in_co mplex_regional_pain.7.aspx

A JOURNEY TO THE LIGHT AND BACK
Sandra L. Arnone

On October 4, 2017, I was sitting at my desk signing off my computer, glad that the day was over. The cast on my right leg felt so heavy, I had only had the cast on for two days due to the Avulsion fracture of the ankle that I suffered a few weeks before on September 22nd which is my birthday. I said oh well, it will heal and I will be fine.

But, as I turned off the computer, I felt like I was falling from my chair and the guy that was behind me caught me. Wow, great reflexes! I started sweating profusely and he noticed this was going on, so he plugs in a little fan to help me. He then said rest here for a minute. I started to hyperventilate and I started to get a pounding headache. I then said where is Ani?

I said that my ride should be here by now. I notice that it was getting harder to breathe and I felt so hot. Now the girl sitting next to me asked me if I had asthma? I told her that I did not have asthma. She thought that I might have been having an anxiety attack? She told me to calm down, and I started to feel my left side go numb, I mean my whole left side from the top of my head to the end of my toes. I started to panic and then I said I think I'm having a stroke?

My friend Monica of 20 years, came over to me and said what's wrong? I said in between breaths, touch my toes. She touched my toes and I could not feel anything. Finally, the office manager said to call 911.

I frantically told Monica I can't feel my left side. Oh God, I can't breathe! She said to me ok calm down the ambulance is coming.

When the paramedics arrived, they realize there was no elevator. They started to strap me into a chair with wheels. As they turn me around, I saw Ani. I yelled; I cannot feel my left side. I am panicked now. The look on her face was like Oh God!

They got me into the ambulance and while taking my vitals, they keep telling me to breathe in through my nose and out my mouth. I could not catch my breath. I told them that I could not feel my left side. They keep telling me to calm down and breathe. I said to myself shit, why aren't they listening to me?

At the hospital there was no bed available, so they parked me in the hallway. At this time, I'm still hyperventilating. It seems like forever before they rolled me into a room.

The doctor came into the room, and immediately calls for a CT scan. Just as quickly I'm rolling in and out of the machine the doctor comes in and said to me, you have a pulmonary embolism and you're only at 60% oxygen and dropping fast.

We need to intubate you now. At this point, it was difficult to talk and breathe, so I ask for a writing pad. I write down no tubes and I said in between breathes-NO TUBES!

The doctor looks worried and confers with two more doctors. My sister walks over to me and says sternly, you have to breathe, you have to do it. I shake my head no-I don't want tubes.

So, the doctor comes over and said okay, we're going to put an oxygen mask that will force air into your lungs forcefully, so I agreed to do that and the nurse complies.

Ani was pacing in the hallway and the look on my son's face was not good. I did not know it then, but they had told my sisters, my chance of making it was slim without doing the intubation.

So, then the doctor said I have one treatment option, it's called tissue plasminogen activator (TPA). He went on to tell me it is a clot-buster medication, a very strong blood thinner, and it has a very serious side effect. It can cause a brain bleed.

This was all he can do to help me to start breathing again. He had to break up the clot that was directly in the middle of my lungs, which was blocking them from letting me get enough oxygen.

So, my sisters said sign it, sign it. I said ok, it's just something they will put in my I.V. if it doesn't work, it doesn't work. I show the doctor my DNR.

He looks at the two other doctors and said nope, not on my watch and cues the nurse. So, at this point, the mask is forcing big bursts of air in my mouth and down my lungs. Something is added to my I.V... I feel myself drift off to sleep, ah nice......

I woke up in the ICU room alone. I rip the oxygen mask off; my throat was so dry. I did not see any water. Then a nurse comes in quickly and said you need that mask and I said wait, now I can breathe and she gives me the little thin oxygen tube and starts taking my vitals. The doctor comes in and I said hey doc I'm all better I can breathe; can I go back to work now? I said half-joking and half-seriously, I hate hospitals. He said now wait a minute and take a minute to tell me how you feel. I said, well, I can breathe okay, but I grab my head and said I have this terrible headache. He told the orderlies to get me to CT scan department stat!

Long story short, I had a Pulmonary embolism, two brain hemorrhages, three strokes, they discovered I had patent foramen ovale (PFO) which is a hole in my heart since birth. I have also had surgery to insert IVF filter, surgery to remove multiple clots from the left side of my body. I saw the light! This was my near-death experience (NDE) or what I call an out of body experience (OBE).

I spent two weeks in the hospital, then I went into a rehab hospital for another two weeks. I had my sister get me out of there against doctors' orders because I could not stand being there. The alarm on the beds and waiting to urinate. No thank you! Not for me!

Six months later I had my cast removed and the Ortho doctor said the bone is healed. I said great, but why is it still painful, swollen and purple? I also had two rounds of physical therapy that did not help me at all.

The PCP that I have seen for the past 10-years told me that I needed to find a new doctor because my case has become too complicated for him to treat me. I did find a new doctor from Upland, CA, and has accepted me and is promising.

My CRPS

I developed complex regional pain syndrome (CRP) from the trauma of the stroke and the avulsion fracture of my left ankle.

In the beginning, none of the doctors were able to tell me why my leg and ankle would not heal? I had gone to a pain management clinic that did confirm I have CRPS.

To date, I have not had any surgeries for my CRPS. I have been offered nerve blocks, but I have refused them so far, due to the fear that they may create more complications for me.

Medications do help me. I am now on a total of 18 medications at this time. Also, the Psych meds that I take have kept me sane.

Another thing that has helped me is the three CRPS support groups that I belong to on Facebook.

Two days after I returned home from the rehab hospital, I woke up next to my Fiancé to find that she had passed away in her sleep during the night. She had her health problems. I believe the stress of me getting sick from the strokes and the CRPS, contributed to her death?

After her death, I had to take care of myself with some help from my sister and some select friends.

Five months later I found a new partner. Her name is Monica and we moved in with each other in April of 2018. She is 41 years old and is also a diabetic.

We are still together, but it is a challenge trying to get her to believe that I am in chronic pain daily. No one believes it, understands it or takes it seriously. I believe it comes with the territory of living in chronic pain.

On July 13, 2018, I had my fourth stroke in the lobby of CVS, while I was going in to pick up my medications.

I have also developed plantar fasciitis in my left foot, so walking has become more and more difficult. I also drive with my left foot and I believe I always will.

Other issues that I have developed are chronic UTI's, I became anemic, antibiotic-resistant, and I have gained substantial weight.

Some of the things that I enjoy doing are swimming, bike riding, and spending time with my grandson named Rhythm Sol.

It's now 2020 and I am back to work again four days a week with doctors' restrictions. I am working in Engineering.

I have gone from a wheelchair to using a walker, to now using a cane. I do okay most days, but I will never run with my grandson born on August 6, 2018, with whom I can walk only a couple of feet.

I am now 49-years old and I have to wear medical dog tags in case of a medical emergency and my DNR is still active.

I think about how my life will end and hopefully on my terms and when I am ready and tired of being in pain.

But who knows? Time will tell!

Thank you for reading my story.

Sandra

IMPRESSIONS OF WELLNESS – DEFINING MY LIFE WITH CRPS
Angi Blake

Being a musician was always my dream. And I was there! I had it, and I DID it! Finally, after a lifetime of working on my craft, I was there. 1994 was going to be my year. 1995 hits, we have more gigs than we know what to do with. We are a group, without the help of roadies. Which only means one thing, pay your dues, and do it yourself. I was incredibly happy to do so.

On, July 7, 1995, we had two gigs in one day. WOW, how incredible. While striking equipment to move, it to the next gig, I hit a speed bump. I was grabbing the microphone bases, (back in the day, they were solid iron) I had placed the one in my right hand down in the truck, and the one in my left hand, I was getting ready to put down. Just then, someone caught my attention to ask a question. BAM, I dropped the base in my left-hand right-on top of my right. My right hand was crushed between two solid iron microphones stand bases, breaking it in three places. A HUGE rush to the hospital, to get it put into a cast. Move on with life. Or, so I thought?

Shortly after my bone was healed, I had a terrible feeling in my hand. With extreme sensitivity to temps, terrible swelling, and sharp pain. My hand burning hot and cold. It was bluish-gray in color, suddenly I noticed the hair growth was just odd. Dark, and grew like mad. (I am a redhead, cannot see my hair on my legs/arms) My nails even changed, brittle, very brittle, and pealed weird like. But they grew crazy long even while brittle. I noticed that stress made everything worse. And boy was I stressed. My music career came to a screeching halt because I couldn't concentrate beyond the pain. All I could do is cry and hold my breath for my next move.

I went first to see my primary care doctor. 'The pain is in your head, there is no way that you can still feel your hand 'pain' now, the bones have healed'. You are fine. This answer wasn't good enough. I knew what I was feeling, and seeing. It was then that I choose to go to see a specialist without the help of insurance. They ran so many tests. Doctor M., at that time, said I don't know what is going on. Something is there, I just don't know what." THAT'S IT? THAT'S ALL I GET? NO MORE RESEARCH? Just take it and go home? I was humiliated. And started second-guessing myself. How could I have something no one believes or can diagnose? Was it in my head after all? NO! I cannot will my hand to swell, turn red and sweat and be hot and cold at the same time. I am not going nuts! But who will believe me? Where do I go from here? I had nothing, just nothing.

Over the next year, I saw nine specialists. From hand doctors, rheumatologists, psychiatrists, neurologists, and pain doctors. All of them had no answers. But the pain continued. It was outrageous pain. Nothing would subside it even in the least bit. All while attempting to keep a job. Each job, I was taking more and more time off. Exhaustion, burning, not sleeping, horrific swelling, and now, hot spots or odd lesions on my hand, as well as the inability able to function and think clearly. I was let go from my favorite job due to the manager thinking I was on something. This would go on for years. Each doctor would give me a new diagnosis. Raynaud's syndrome, Tendonitis, C-6, and C-7 nerve entrapment. Thoracic outlet syndrome (TOS), fibromyalgia, and from one doctor, even 'some sort of psychosis'. My ex-husband had enough of it all, told me I was crazy and that he was leaving. This destroyed me. He attempted to take my son from me, calling me unfit. My world was destroyed.

With all this going on, I continued my life. Working, taking time off work to go see a specialist, being told I'm nuts or have some bizarre condition and no one could help. In 1999, I met the love of my life. Being fearful, I explained everything to him about what was going on in my life and yet, he stuck around. In 2001 I married the crazy man who pledged his life to me. He said 'We WILL find an answer'. My husband was a 20-year veteran. With that, little did I know came insurance. Even making the long drudge to the base often, they still had no idea what was happening. But they tried. I had numerous x-rays, blood tests, MRI's, all the things that would tell them absolutely nothing. Then I was sent to a new pain Doctor, Doctor. P., who said to me "What you have is reflex sympathetic dystrophy (RSD) and I cannot help you. There is NO cure. And really, it's so misunderstood, no one can do anything for you. But I will send you to PT, perhaps desensitization will help. You mean to tell me it is 2003, we have crazy technology, put people on the moon, and you can't fix this? Physical therapy made me hurt worse than I was already hurting. They manipulated me, moved me, even iced my hand. Then warmed it in a blanket. This was torture. Worse than I've been through before. The physical therapist sent me back to the pain doctor and all he did was ordered more PT and gave me Gabapentin. The dose started pretty low, then gradually increased over a couple of years I saw him. Finally, a full 80 lbs., heavier, I was on 3600 mg of Gabapentin. THERE MUST BE ANOTHER WAY?

I lived like this for years, and miserable. Still working, still getting odd looks from coworkers for my weight gain. Still having bosses that don't believe my pain. Thinking I'm just lazy.

In 2013, I had enough. I couldn't work. Showering hurts, and it takes all my energy. Just breathing some days is all I can do. My whole being went downhill. The pain doctor that I was seeing, Doctor H, who was doing stellate ganglion blocks (SGB) on me. He would put me under, move my larynx and my esophagus and put a needle with medication directly into my sympathetic nerve. He did this procedure approximately 30 times over a couple of years. In time, pushing my larynx over to administer the block, changed my vocal quality. Now I couldn't reach the notes anymore. This is all I was able to keep from my prior music-life, and now, he has destroyed that. Then depression set in and it was hard. I couldn't find the motivation to get up in the morning. And I would say to myself, "what's the use?" Doctor H., said, "you have depression, you need to see a psychologist and I will not see you anymore." FABULOUS! Now the only guy who sort of knew what was happening to me bailed. What do I do now? My depression hit an all-time low. Even my husband was worried.

With the help of a friend, we found another pain doctor. The doctor's location was close to my work. So, I could take lunch, and just see this doctor. At, my first appointment, he reviewed all my records and said you've had everything done.

You may want to think about a spinal cord stimulator (SCS). He gave me a pamphlet, and gave me pain meds, then sent me on my way. Sounds crazy, implant something that buzzed my pain away. I thought Doctor P was nuts. But I'm done with this.

2014 came along, and I could not work anymore. All my attempts became futile. The pain was great, the brain fog was destroying how I felt about myself. I couldn't remember anything. My employer just let me go and said you aren't an asset if you can't perform your job, and remember things. So much for an income. I went back to see the Doctor P., and weirdly enough, he left the practice and had a new guy in his place, Doctor D., I spoke with him regarding the stimulator I previously discussed with the Doctor P., and he said they would set me up for a trial. Regarding the pain meds, the more meds you are on, the more you will need, they will

44

never be enough, your receptors are broken because of the pain meds. Well, that's great news… UGH! I opted, against my judgment, I finally applied for disability. It was November 2014, I have a real problem, I've been paying into this for many, many years. I should be granted disability insurance. Gave me a moment of peace, of mind.

January 2, 2015, was my SCS trial to evaluate the effectiveness. During this time, I was able to move a little more. I still had pain, but it was at a 7 instead of the 9/10 that I was living with. On January 5, 2015, the temporary stimulator was removed. The Doctor said it should be within three weeks to have the permanent unit implanted. Unfortunately, the doctor's office was very behind, therefore my case was put on hold. They forgot to get the authorization, and they weren't sure how to request the authorization, for a neurosurgeon. The process took four months instead of the promised three weeks.

On May 26, 2015, Doctor W., met me at the surgery center in Phoenix and implanted the stimulator. The paddle leads were put into my neck, and I had to wear a neck brace for six weeks while the scar tissue built up around the leads. After 10-days, the stimulator was turned on and working. The pain subsided and I lost 40 lbs., over the year that it was working. Yay…

However, bad news, I was denied my disability. Things started getting turned off one at a time. I robbed Peter to pay Paul, and Peter was running out of money. This went on for years. Took me four and a half years to get approved for disability. I almost lost my home three times. My husband did NOT fight for this country for 20-years of his life to lose his home due to his wife was sick! After three tries and four and a half years, we went to trial, and I won my disability case. While this was great news, when the funds were put into my account, they did not ask if we wanted taxes taken out. Therefore, the whole sum was deposited, leaving us a HUGE amount to answer for at tax time. Leaving us to owe quite a bit for 2018. I later found out, I needed to submit form W-4V (Voluntary Withholding Request) to my local Social Security Office. And funds will be taken out of my monthly disability check. Hopefully, we will NOT owe for 2019. I later went on to find out that I could have printed out, and given my attorney an article from the Social Security Administration regarding disability insurance. This article effective date was October 20, 2003. It was stating where CRPS is, in fact, a qualifying factor for disability insurance.

Documents needed to prove it from the physician, including how much time off you would need to take care of yourself. As well as a documented list of all your medications and doctor's prognosis.

By 2016, I had lost enough weight, that my generator/battery pack that was implanted in my back, had flipped over. The doctors had no other option than to surgically do a pocket revision, and move the generator/battery pack to my hip. At this time, I saw a different surgeon/doctor. The doctor I was seeing was not doing surgeries at that time. Doctor B., the surgeon who moved my generator/battery pack, followed up with me a week after surgery. He said "slight" redness around the left side of the incision but looks good. This was August 15, 2016. By August 21, 2016, I woke with no therapy at all, had extreme pain, the first year all over again. I phoned the doctor, my doctor, my primary care, and Medtronic (the manufacturer of SCS). Finally, I have another appointment with Doctor B., and Medtronic's. After the last surgery, the whole left side of the battery lead was not working. Medtronic gave me two new programs and set an appointment up for September 9, 2016, to surgically go in and reconnect the wires. Long as I had my hand on my hip, and pressed hard, I had therapy. Well, that's inconvenient!

By this time, I was getting weekly Ketamine infusions. When I went for my first one, the doc was Doctor P. He knew my history, and was anxious to see how Ketamine would work, for my pain and the depression. He asked if I knew the basis of my depression. Apparently, it's not obvious to a doctor that you have extreme pain, and no one knows how to help would possibly lead to depression. Not to mention waking in the morning wondering where you will be when the bad one hits, and how bad is bad going to be.

By September 5, 2016, I woke in even more extreme pain. It felt like the wires were being pulled from my hip to my neck. There was a large moving lump on my neck. HORRIBLE, HORRIBLE PAIN. By the following day, I was calling everyone to find out what was going on. I had emergency surgery on September 7, 2016, to reconnect wires and put an extension in at my hip. Doctor B., had me stay in the hospital with six bags of IV antibiotics. I had a slight infection at the incision site, and he still proceeded to go in and fix the stimulator. The hospital did a CT scan to pacify me, they still had no idea what was going on.

On September 14, 2016, I had a follow up with Doctor B., to do a wound check. He said it all looks fine, still no idea about the lump. After a one-month follow-up with my regular pain doctor, he had no idea about it, he sent me to the ER for the lump. My doctor was fearful of what it could be. At the ER, I ran into Doctor H., who said, he did a CT scan, then said "I've done my job, there is nothing wrong with you, if you want meds, go home, you have them there" FINE! Looks like I will never get help. I'm doomed to hurt for the rest of my life and have docs that are in denial of what I am telling them.

When I returned to my normal pain doctor, he attempted to aspirate. There was no fluid at that time. He spoke with Doctor B., and at that time,

Doctor B., admitted, there must have been someone in the operating room (OR) that introduced an infection.

By October 4, 2016, my husband rushed me to the ER (this time a different one) the lump has erupted, the infection was coming out. I was transferred to a hospital in Phoenix because they have a Neurosurgeon on staff. Strangely, that Neurosurgeon, was the same Surgeon who implanted my SCS on May 26, 2015. The hospital kept me for four days after my surgery to remove the Medtronic unit. At that time, I was given Ciprofloxacin 750 mg. This medication attacked my muscles. Made my recovery at home even more difficult. It felt like I had been immobilized for months.

I couldn't lift my arms. Yet, still, I burned beyond belief. I couldn't even feed myself. I couldn't lift my arms. By now, I was in extreme pain without the stimulator. My swelling was worse than I've ever seen it. The cramping was horrific, and now, sharp, burning pain everywhere. Again, I felt like I went back to the beginning.

By now, my regular pain doctor that I loved working with, had moved on to a new facility. My one month follow up was with a doctor that was horrible. He had no answers. Again, no answers. What is wrong with the community that doctors don't know what to do? My follow-up with the surgeon that removed my SCS, said I could get it back in a couple of months. The infection had to be gone for good. They made it clear at the time, they don't know why the last surgery was performed while I had signs of an infection. That should NEVER have been done. The infection started at my hip, moved up the wires, and manifested in my neck. My SCS was finally re-implanted on December 20, 2016. However, this time, on the left side. No, the right side that I have CRPS in. My God, how much can I go through?

On May 3, 2018, I woke with intermittent therapy. Depending on how I hold my head. I placed a call to the doctor. Then he sent me to the Neurosurgeon in Phoenix again. He stated it should be easy, like 'taking off and on a glove and giving me an upgraded Medtronic system. Well, that sounds promising. On June 8, 2018, the surgery party again. He noted that the wires were broken at the neck. He replaced the whole system and the leads on the left side because of previous infection and scar tissue. It does not function well as I hoped, I get 30/70 satisfaction depending on the day and circumstances. I'm disappointed, however, I guess any type of relief is good to an CRPS patient. But the unit does not work as well as the first one, due to all the scar tissue from multiple surgeries. Still the pain level is an 8/9 out of 10. Then another pocket revision. WOW! Seriously? On November 19, 2018, I could not breathe due to the pain from my battery pack. It was implanted under my bra strap. Another crap storm from the insurance company. Everyone was pointing fingers saying no one asked for authorization, it fell through the cracks... blah, blah, blah. After all, they aren't in the pain. FINALLY, on April 4, 2019, I had to have surgery to move the generator/battery pack. Unfortunately, she discovered that it wedged itself under my shoulder blade. Thus, making it hard to breathe. However, she noticed that I still was not moving my arm the way she thought it should move because of the burning pain, so she decided that I needed another lead. A different kind of lead. This time, she implanted a subcutaneous lead going up to my C-4 and moved my battery pack farther to the left close to my side. Doctor S., attempted to do this surgery with a local. I can still feel the knife cutting my back.

By the time the surgery was over, I was crying uncontrollably, I was in horrific pain. I laid in the hospital room, just wanting to die. Over the years, I've lost so much. My life, my livelihood, my career, my music, ambition ability to conquer life. Loss of friends, employment. What was I

49

left with? Pain, burning atrophy in my wrist, osteoporosis, crappy teeth, low self-esteem and 14 7" scars all up and down my back. Not to mention the pain no one believes understands or avoids you to not hear about it. The medications that are endless and all the crazy surgeries. I felt like all the medical field wanted to do was "dartboard" therapy. Between ablations, nerve blocks, and hypnosis. All failing, and destructive to who I was. They had no idea what was wrong with me, and so quick and easy to jump to "It's all in your head". I was put on some crazy medications. Sumatriptan, Ultram 50 mg, Lyrica, Celebrex, Tegretol, Soma, Klonopin, Effexor XR 7 (for depression), Motrin 800 mg 3x/day, Darvocet, Tizanidine HCL 6 mg, Ketamine Nasal Spray Quinine, Oxymorphone Hydrochloride Extended-Release 20 mg (PAIN), Cyclobenzaprine hydrochloride 5 mg (muscle spasms), a topical cream AB1-KETAMINE 10%, Gabapentin 6%, Diclofenac 3%, Baclofen 2%, Lidocaine 2% cream, however, this was crazy expensive, and the insurance was not going to pay for it. Neurontin 3600 mg which made me had even more brain fog than usual, and gain bad weight. They need a new dartboard to throw their darts at. What they were trying was NOT working. Even making it worse in some cases.

In October 2019, my Doctor D., said, "Enough of this". I'm not putting you through another failed surgery. I believe the best way to go is an intrathecal pain pump filled with Dilaudid. As of October 25, 2019, my pain doctor implanted the pain pump after a 'successful' trial on September 24, 2019. The flow has been increased twice so far. First time by 50%, the second time by 40%. He indicated that one more increase and we should be 'there'. At the moment, I am still on Oxycodone 10mg, Morphine ER 30mg 2x/day, and Ketamine Nasal spray. I still get Ketamine Infusions to help control the pain as well. I have another planned surgery on February 14, 2020, to remove one of the leads and my generator/battery pack. When the doctor went in and filled the pain pump, he used the fluoroscope

50

and noted that the lead that was last implanted by Doctor S., at my C-4 level, has slid down to my T-6 level. At the moment, that lead that slipped is directed diagonally on my right shoulder blade and causes huge pain issues. In addition to what I already have. Hoping this next surgery will fix that.

From the beginning, my CRPS has spread. From the middle finger to my shoulder, across to my neck, and down between my shoulder blades. I also and effected on my right ankle, and now, it has spread to my intestines. For me, it feels like I've been soaking my arm in ice water for a couple of hours, which set off the fire pain, then it feels like I am being stabbed with ice picks. It is relentless. Then, there are horrific cramps where I cannot move. The prolonged pain is constant, pins and needles, stabbing, burning and miserable. I even have days that when I attempt to lay down to get rest, just the weight of the sheet will send me through the roof. How can this be?

My doctor explained it as your nerve is like a fire hose turned on full blast. When you let go of the hose, the hose flops uncontrollably everywhere.

CRPS has changed my life, my outlook and my dreams. I still am passionate about my music, however, in the beginning, too many SGB have ruined that for me. Friends do not always want to hear "how you are doing," even though they ask. Doctors don't know it all. No matter how well educated, they appear to be. We have the disease, not the doctors, they don't know what is going on they are trying to help without complete knowledge. Listening to your body, and not pushing yourself is the best thing you can do. Just because you feel better one day does not mean that you have to rule the world. You will pay for it. CRPS is not in your head. If a doctor tells you this, find another doctor.

What I have learned. Throughout my journey, I've learned that Vitamin C helps the radical spread of this disease. I take 1000 mg with each meal, and Extended-Release Vitamin C before bedtime. I've learned recently, if you do surgery, an epidural nerve block before, during and after surgery can help the CRPS from spreading. I've learned that I have CRPS but, it does not have me. We are in control of our outlook, no matter how hard that is. We must train ourselves to find a bright spot for our mental health. Our bodies are trying to kill us, we don't have to let it happen. Your frame of mind is KEY. I've learned that although I am in extreme pain, the best thing I can do is communicate with people who don't understand. We MUST find a cure, if not for us, for the children who have this disastrous disease. No matter what people say, do not, under any condition use ice, which makes it 10,000 worse. I've learned to find someone you can vent to. This person should not ALWAYS be your spouse. Resentment can come easily that way. We aren't in it alone. You just need to find that person. No matter how hard it is, strength does come from within. I smile through the tears because I need that for my mental health. There is no cure, I'm stuck with this for always and forever. I strive to find good in every day, or I'm just miserable. And that is not fair to those around me, especially my husband.

Because of my experiences over the years, and the way I was treated, I started a project very near and dear to my heart. I make hospital comfort bears. I send these bears out with all the information on CRPS, as well as a disc drive to put your information on, and a bracelet that says ALERT, Complex Regional Pain Syndrome. I would never want anyone treated like I was in the beginning. It is a lonely place to be.

BEHIND THE SMILE
Tavia Palmer

My name is Tavia Palmer. I am 44-years old, and in March of 2015, I was working for Uber. One day, while I was out driving for Uber, I was involved in a car accident and hit by a drunk driver.

During this car accident, I suffered a head injury, which led to debilitating pain in my head. I kept telling the doctors it felt like somebody had poured gasoline on my brain, and lit me on fire. I can't stand anything touching my scalp, wear a baseball cap, or glasses. It was so bad I couldn't even stand having my head laying on a pillow.

I kept getting diagnosed with migraines, and they threw every migraine medication at me to help treat my pain. I kept telling them, "Migraine medications are not working!" In May 2018, I finally opted to get a spinal cord stimulator (SCS) implant to treat my pain.

Shortly after the implant surgery, the pain traveled into my feet. The pain was so bad I couldn't walk. My feet, ankles, and calves started to swell up. The pain was a deep burning yet, cold at the same time. When I would get up and walk, it felt like I was walking on glass, and having sharp nails driven into my feet. I have been primarily bedridden for the last almost five years of my life.

Trying to get pain management or find a doctor who knows what I have been dealing with was nearly impossible. When I lived in Oklahoma, I was assigned a new Medtronic representative to help me program SCS. I told him what my symptoms were, and he asked me if I had ever heard of complex regional pain syndrome (CRPS) or if anyone has mentioned that I may have it?

For years, I had been searching for an answer to my pain. When I looked it up, the list of symptoms for CRPS, it was spot on to my pain. I had my answer, and the relief came over me, but this relief was short-lived. I finally had an answer, but it had the worst outcome. Having an answer became the next exhausting fight of my life.

Since I moved to Texas, the doctors advised me I needed psychiatric help. I've met with pain specialists who told me my case was too complex for them to treat. After being disappointed by doctors, again and again, I turned to alcohol to help relieve my pain.

Several times, I have ended up in the hospital after drinking too much alcohol, just trying to numb the pain. Getting narcotics is nearly impossible. Taking Narcotics is the only thing to knock out my pain. After moving to Houston, Texas, I found a Ketamine clinic and had six Ketamine infusions, which were very helpful. The problem I had is, the clinic does not bill the insurance company, and trying to get the insurance company to pay for it is difficult. So, I had to spend $8,000 of my own money only to be right back where I started when I couldn't do it anymore.

Nobody seems to have an answer for me. I finally got an official diagnosis of CRPS by my pain management doctor in Houston. The doctor treating me severed our relationship after one of my bouts with alcohol. I had ordered a copy of the medical records. After reviewing the medical records, I found that the doctor never answered the reason for my drinking. He only recorded my mental state.

I tried to explain that if they treated my pain, all my other issues would have gone away. Anyone suffering from the pain of CRPS for over five years would be depressed and have a sense of hopelessness.

I feel the medical community should be there for us when we are sick, but it has failed me and so many others suffering from this disease. They call CRPS the suicide disease, and I cannot say that I have not been there many times since the day of my accident. I have lost friends; my relationship with my family has changed because they don't understand my pain. No one should ever have to live with something like this. It is inhumane!

Remember, CRPS patients are just waiting for an answer. So, we have to hold on and take things one day at a time.

MY JOURNEY WITH CRPS: FROM HELL TO HEALING
Tracey Morales

Hi, my name is Tracey, I'm 49-years-old; married with two daughters. My complex regional pain syndrome (CRPS) story started on January 18, 1998, when a toy V-Tech computer fell on my left foot, fracturing two toes, and crushing the MT joints (toe knuckles). After two weeks, I knew something was wrong, my pain was much worse, and the bruising was going up my foot.

So, I saw a podiatrist, who by the second appointment, on February 10th, diagnosed me with CRPS. He sent me to a vascular surgeon who confirmed the diagnosis with a triple-phase bone scan. They referred to an anesthesiologist to have a sympathetic nerve block which confirmed the CRPS, and if it would help relieve my symptoms, which at this point were extreme pain and sensitivity. I couldn't wear a sock on. The skin discoloration at this point was now up to my knee, and I had a temperature difference between my feet and legs.

I experienced six sympathetic nerve blocks and six days of hospitalization with an epidural catheter in six weeks. All worked, but wore off in 24-hours or less, CRPS came back fighting, worse after each treatment, I found out. My leg was now on fire, but ice-cold, and so discolored from my groin to my toes, it looked like someone colored my leg with a magic marker. We decided to do a sympathectomy, done on March 18th, exactly two months after the initial injury. On the morning of my surgery, my doctor said my big toe was getting gangrene, even though repeated vascular ultrasounds showed significant blood flow.

The sympathectomy worked, I went into remission for four years. I went back to work, got married, and had my second daughter. When she was two-years-old, she had her tonsils removed, and I stayed in the hospital with her. I fell asleep in the bed with her, not realizing that my foot was up against the footboard. I woke up the next morning, stood-up, and the CRPS was back. I could not put any weight on my foot without excruciating pain. I saw my doctor that week, and he confirmed my CRPS was back. My only real option was taking medications because the sympathetic nerve was no longer there. They had removed about 12 inches of the nerve during the surgery four years prior. The nerve had started to regrow at the base of my spinal cord about a 1/4 of an inch, that very tiny growth was enough for it to come back in my left leg even though the sympathetic nerve was no longer connected.

The CRPS ended up going full-body over the next few years. I was bedridden 95% of the time. I tried more nerve blocks, lidocaine infusions over the years, as the nerve grew more, but nothing worked. I was on countless medications, but it continued to get worse.

In 2005, I spoke with a friend from high school. She suggested I make an appointment with a doctor that she worked with, who was doing experimental Ketamine infusions. So, I made an appointment with Doctor S., a neurologist from Philadelphia, PA. I had to wait a year and a half for my appointment. I started the infusions in January 2007. I initially went for 10-days, then for three days every two to three months for booster infusions for a period over 10-years.

For the first eight-years, the treatments worked pretty well, and it helped to reduce my pain down to a 5-6 on the pain scale. It also reversed my full-body spread, back to just being in my left leg. In the last two years, the Ketamine stopped working for me. My pain came back again, to an 8-10, and my CRPS spread into my right leg. I could not see spending more money if the treatments were not working anymore. I stopped. My last infusion was in December 2016.

At this point, I was very frustrated, my pain medication was up to a 200-mcg Fentanyl patch every two days, and I was taking Opana (oxymorphone hydrochloride) for any breakthrough pain. I could not wear a sock again, and just having a sheet touch my legs caused excruciating pain. My oldest daughter was getting married in October 2017. I had no idea how I would make it through the four-day event, or even to the wedding itself.

In early April, I received an e-mail through my Awareness Items store that I do design for, from a man interested in a ribbon that I designed for CRPS. I saw that the e-mail said OSKA at the top, after speaking with him I asked what OSKA was, and he told me all about it. I quickly decided that I needed to try this device.

In April 2017, I started using the Oska Pulse Device, and that has brought my pain down to almost nothing. It's helping with so many different symptoms, and I have been able to take back my life and do the things I love to do again.

I am getting better relief from the Oska Pulse Device than I did from the infusions. My pain was an 8-9-10+ on a bad day, the CRPS was spreading into my right leg, a good day my pain was a 5-6, with the infusions. Now my pain today is a 1-2 on a good day, and a three on a bad day, which is rare. The weather does not bother me anymore. I used to get three to five migraines every week. I have not had one since I started using Oska. The shocking and electrocution type of pain I would feel in my leg has stopped. I have not had a flare since June 2017, and I no longer have swelling or discoloration of the skin. As of January 12, 2020, I stopped using the Fentanyl patch, which I was on for 18-years.

I have a 20-year-old daughter; who suffers from POTS (Postural Orthostatic Tachycardia Syndrome), EDS, Endometriosis, and TMJ. She has had symptoms since kindergarten, but her doctors finally diagnosed her at age 14.

It is difficult when your child has an illness, especially when you have an illness with similar symptoms. There are pros and cons to this. Pros: I can be more sympathetic, understanding, and supporting. Cons: I know how horrible she feels. Being her parent, and knowing how tough things are, and not being able to fix it, is awful.

Thankfully, the Oska Pulse Device helps her too. Now she is going to college full-time and working two part-time jobs.

I have found some good out of the bad. I had started drawing awareness pictures to keep my mind off my pain. That led to a Facebook Artwork page, and a store on Zazzle, where my designs are available on T-shirts, Leggings, Jewelry, Sneakers, and many other items. I have over 35 different illnesses items. I have made several donations with my royalties, and plan to make more as time goes on.

Thank you for taking the time to read my CRPS story. We need a cure for this monster; it's taken so much from so many. Please spread the word about this horrific Illness.

Tracey

BITTEN - A STORM FROM WITHIN
Deb Leach

My Complex Regional Pain Syndrome (CRPS) journey started simply. The day started like any other day. This simple start to the day, has never ended.

I recently had been laid off from work, and the days of looking for a new job were long. To fill a void, I decided to volunteer at our local SPCA. I adored being at the shelter. I couldn't wait to wake up in the morning and rush to the shelter. I was spending more time volunteering than actually looking for a job. I loved everything about it. I did a little bit of everything, walked dogs, washed dog and cat bowls, did laundry and oftentimes swept the floor. As time went on, I felt more comfortable being in the cat room. I fostered numerous cats, bringing them home made it easier for me to pursue a new job but also volunteer. My active boys even enjoyed playing with the kittens and cats I brought home to foster. It became a family affair.

Eventually I found a part time position where I could work in the morning and volunteer in the afternoon. It was such a fulfilling time for me. It wasn't unusual for me to be at the shelter on the weekend. This particular day when my CRPS journey began as any other day, it was March 31, 2013 Easter Sunday. The shelter was closed to the general public for adoptions but was open for volunteers. It was perfect, I could go and help without the distraction of the public coming in. I came into the shelter and one of the first cats I would socialize this day was a Bengal cat. Bengal cats are half domestic house cats and half Asian Leopards. They are beautiful and elegant in every way. By nature, they do not like to be caged. This cat's name was Daisy. She was just beautiful. She has the most stunning eyes! I had held her several times previous to this, she was always calm and eager to get out of the cage. I was known at the shelter as a senior volunteer, I had worked there several years and was committed to helping animals.

At the time I was holding Daisy, I was speaking to the director, he was commenting on how beautiful she was, we made some small talk and he left to go out of the cat area. But instead of just walking out, he slammed the door. No sooner did the metal of the door hit the metal of the door jamb Daisy reacted. She bit me with all of her might. It was so quick; my brain did not even have time to process what happened. She jumped back into her cage and stared at the wall. Almost as if she knew what she had done. It took me a few moments to figure out what just happened. I first checked to make sure Daisy was ok and locked her cage and then went to the bathroom. There was not a drop of blood, I barely even saw a mark. I washed where I thought she had bitten me, clearly, I was fine! Or I thought.

Other volunteers started to come into the shelter as I had, I let them know what happened and continued to volunteer for another hour. I needed to go home, I was having dinner at my sister's house and needed to cook a few side dishes. My finger was sore, but there weren't any signs to me that something was wrong. We left to go to my sister's house. There was a little red mark on the top of my finger which was the only outward sign that something was wrong.

During dinner, my finger started to swell and ache. It became grossly red. At that moment I looked down and saw how red it was, I knew! I knew it was infected. I needed to go to the Emergency Room.

Unfortunately, we had to drive my son back to college which would be around a two-hour round-trip ride. For certain this was the longest two hours of my life thus far. My finger now was throbbing, it was very swollen and hurt unbelievably.

We finally made it to the Emergency Room, the doctor on call really did not think it was much of a concern. After a few hours at the hospital he just gave me an antibiotic and sent me home with a prescription. Now, my finger was beyond painful and even more swollen.

It was late when we got home, I had to go to work the next day. During the night I couldn't sleep because my elbow hurt. I woke up, took a shower and got ready for work. I said goodbye to my husband and told him I would get the prescription filled for the antibiotic at lunch. I started to drive to work but something inside of me told me to drive back to the Emergency Room. I am not sure why I made this decision and why I felt the need to go, but it was an overwhelming feeling

I let them know that I was just there the night before and that I couldn't sleep because of the pain. I found out that if the infection had gone up my arm and was just about at my shoulder. I was told that if it reached past my shoulder that they wouldn't be able to help me, that the infection had gone too far. Fortunately, I made that decision to go to the emergency room that day instead of work. I would spend the next five days in the hospital on intravenous antibiotics (IV). This would be the start of a constant infection for the next three years. The infection would go dormant while on antibiotics but once off the antibiotics the infection would surface. I became allergic to about 10 antibiotics over the course of this on/off of infections.

During this cycle, I would be hospitalized for weeks at a time on IV antibiotics. One time leaving with a PICC line and doing antibiotic treatments at home. While on the PICC line, nurses would come to check in to see how I was doing, on the first occasion the nurse came and used the PICC line to take blood. I thought it was the neatest thing.

She left and almost immediately my arm hurt. I did not say anything, I thought it would go away. I went to work the next day and couldn't raise my arm. I knew something wasn't right and called the nursing company that was assigned to my care while on the PICC line, I was told to go to the ER. I went and found that I had two very large clots on my vein. The PICC line was removed and I spent a week in the hospital as they tried to find out why I made a clot so quickly and got the IV antibiotics I needed. I left with another PICC line in the opposite arm.

I went to work, hid the PICC line and tried to be as strong as I could. I wouldn't let the nurses take blood from the PICC line now, but even with not doing that I made another clot on the new PICC line. I had to give myself Lovenox shots in my stomach as well as take Warfarin. It was daunting, trying to work, trying not to think how much pain I was in. I did not want my husband or sons to know how really bad my hand was hurting. I felt it was my burden and did not want others to be affected by it. The only people who really knew the extent of the pain were my doctors and myself. I had withdrawn from friends and family functions. I wasn't doing my best at work. It is hard to work and have relationships when all you can think about is the pain. The pain I was experiencing controlled everything, even at times sweating because of the pain. I have learned techniques on how to divert my brain to think about pain. I tap my foot or move my finger; it is a diversion to take my mind off of it. This pain is like no other I have experienced. I describe it as a chainsaw buzzing in my hand. That description is still how I feel seven years after the incident. Not sure if you can imagine having a chainsaw buzzing in any part of your body for a moment let alone seven years.

By now I had finished the antibiotics and the PICC line was removed. The doctors did not know the reason why I had made clots so quickly that answer would come six months later. I was tested and retested and checked and rechecked for numerous clotting disorders. I was taking blood thinners and shooting Lovenox into my stomach still. It wasn't until I was safely allowed to stop these that the Hematologist was able to find out that I had a very rare clotting disorder called Protein S Deficiency, type 2. This disorder means I clot super-fast. I had never heard of this disease before.

I did go through a period of time where I doubted, I had this disease and thought that the doctors did not have a clue! How could all these things be happening to one person?

Now that I was on antibiotics it was evident that I was now unable to move my finger. When the cat had bitten me, it had severed nerves, tendons and ligaments. I wasn't aware of the amount of damage that happened on that fateful day. During the three years of infection, my finger, hand and arm were in constant pain. The kind of pain that makes it unbearable to think, the kind of pain that wakes you from a sound sleep, the kind of pain no one should have to endure.

I had never been through an injury like this before so I did not know what to expect. I had always been active and somewhat healthy. I had recently been diagnosed with Rheumatoid Arthritis. But this pain did not compare to any other I had ever experienced. I did not know the torn nerves and tendons caused this much pain. There wasn't a moment where my hand/arm did not hurt. I couldn't sleep, I couldn't concentrate, I couldn't function. I thought it was due to the infection and that the infection had not cleared and was causing undue pain.

I decided to contact a hand surgeon to see if the bite had caused more damage than the ER had explained. I remember my first visit with the surgeon very clearly, we met and I described what had happened and the issues I was having, she examined my hand and x-rays and told my husband and I that she was diagnosing me with CRPS in October of 2013. We left in the car and both my husband and I thought she was nuts! I had never heard of CRPS before and she had to be wrong.

With increasing pain and lack of sleep I made another appointment with another doctor. I was hoping for a different outcome.

This hand surgeon's approach to my lack of mobility was to use a fixator device to my hand and it would need it to be cranked every day. This device had two screws into my bone and a device on the outside that had a little knob to turn. It made sense; this device would loosen the stiff joint. Still debating my CRPS diagnosis, we did surgery to apply this device and daily it was cranked. The pain from cranking this machine was enormous.

But since it was a limited issue, I continued. Eventually after a month of cranking and a period of rest the device was removed. To my horror it did not work at all. My hand hurt more my finger would not move. Nothing had changed. I decided to get another opinion.

My next hand surgeon meeting was much like the first, I was told I had nerve damage, a torn tendon, but more importantly I had CRPS. By now I was experiencing constant pain, my skin had turned shiny and my mobility was limited. This time my husband and I got into the car and started to really Google about CRPS. I educated myself and what I found out online and made one final appointment to see a well-known hand surgeon.

I went to the appointment with the last hand surgeon and was told I had CRPS along with tendon, nerve damage and a neuroma but he would be able to help. That began the first of numerous surgeries on my hand. And it was the day that I was convinced I had CRPS.

By now after three years, the infection had planted itself in my bone. On an MRI it was evident, but the surgeon thought instead of infection it was Rheumatoid Arthritis that had invaded my bone, he decided that a joint replacement would be best. Hoping for mobility and less pain I thought it was a great idea. And at the time I did not know it was infected still. I thought he knew what he was doing.

I had the joint replacement, it lasted less than three months, it was a huge mistake. My finger was horribly infected. I scheduled surgery to have the joint replacement removed and a biopsy to find the bacteria strain. The bacteria came back as Lugenesis. A resistant-bacteria. One that is hard to get rid of.

After this discovery, the surgeon and I discussed scheduling an amputation. I couldn't wrap my head around an amputation. It seemed so drastic, so horrible. A ray resection amputation was scheduled for April 12, 2016. All the while my CRPS has been out of control. Losing more and more mobility, sleep was non-existent. Work was impossible.

I remember clearly the day the bandages came off and looked at what was now my new hand. I nearly fainted, I couldn't look at my hand. Four fingers instead of five. I was worried that people would stare at my hand, I felt incomplete. I was worried my children would think differently of me. I would hide my hand at all times, keeping it behind my back or under a table. I did not want people to stare. After years of living with it, I no longer think that way. I have gotten used to it. I hope when I meet people that after telling my story that they would understand and not stare.

My three-year battle with the bone infection is gone, for the first time in three years, I felt better. I weigh about 100 pounds now. Having the infection made me feel sick and eating wasn't a top priority. Now that the infection was gone and my fight to feel better was now my focus. I started with the constant unrelenting pain.

I mostly thought that the pain was from the infection, but once the infection was gone and the source of the infection was gone, the pain was even more heightened. I had a pain management specialist nearly from the time I was diagnosed with CRPS, but not only from CRPS but also from Rheumatoid Arthritis and now Lupus. Since being bitten, I have developed many autoimmune diseases. Rheumatoid Arthritis, Lupus, Sjogren's, Raynaud's, Hashimoto, Protein S Deficiency and CRPS. These auto-immune diseases are not linked to my accident or CRPS, I had signs of these diseases prior to the accident.

My CRPS by now was my sole focus, it was unrelenting. I can't remember the last time I slept through the night, I can't remember the last time my hand was able to snuggle under the sheets, I can't remember the last time I was able to stick my hand into a pocket, or into a glove. I can't shake anyone's hand; I can't open a door or a jar. I can't pet my animals; I have not been able to hold my husband's hand and I can barely crochet. Crocheting has always been my stress reliever; it kept my mind off of how bad I was feeling.

Since the pain was out of control my pain management doctor suggested I go and see a pain doctor that specializes in CRPS. I made the appointment and again he assessed whether or not I had CRPS, he was the first doctor to take a temperature of both of my hands. After telling me I had CRPS he talked about a device, a spinal cord stimulator (SCS) which would greatly relieve my pain.

I listened and it sounded awesome. By this time, I had been on opioid pain medicine for a while. My family was worried, with opioids flooding the news every day, they were worried I would be another statistic. I was excited to hear about the SCS device and how it could relieve my pain. But now the pain had started to travel and it was getting harder and harder to hide my despair with the pain. The doctor said it would really make a difference. So, in October of 2017 I scheduled to have surgery to have the SCS implanted. He said he would have two wires implanted because he knew it would spread and that way, I wouldn't need another procedure, From the beginning it did not relieve the pain as he said. Yes, it worked but maybe it took 10% percent of the pain away. If I turned the device up higher, it would feel as though I was being electrocuted, so I left it very low.

I was really devastated by the lack of relief this device gave. I had tried several nerve blocks and numerous prescription opioid pain medications all in the attempts to relieve the pain. Every day seemed daunting just trying to make the pain go away. I learned to distract myself. I started to have episodes where I was blacking out. I literally would either be driving, watching tv, working at work and I would black out. I told my general doctor because of the frequency of them and my safety. She gave me the name of a neurologist to see if there was an issue. I never put the blackout periods and the SCS together, never thought there was a relationship between the two.

The SCS stopped giving me any relief, even 10 percent. I told the pain management doctor every visit, it isn't working, I need to up my pain meds. One day I saw him and he told me that I need to go to downtown Philadelphia to a Neurosurgeon who specializes in CRPS and SCS. Immediately I thought, what an inconvenience, to go down to the city, take time off of work and would have to involve my husband driving me.

I went back another time to the pain management doctor and he asked if I had made the appointment, I hadn't. He insisted.

So, with the final nudge I made the appointment. My appointment was a few days before Christmas. We met and told him my current situation. And told him that the spinal cord stimulator was not working. I also let him know that I was blacking out.

The neurosurgeon gave me a speech about a lot of people coming to see him saying their SCS did not work but, in actuality they do, they are not using them properly or don't want them anymore. I looked straight at him and told him, mine doesn't work!

He ordered 12 x-rays of my spine, neck and back. He was checking the placement of the stimulator and wires. I got the x-rays done on December 22nd. I received a call from his office the next day, asking me to come in the doctor needed to see me. I had not looked at the report yet, so I did not know the urgency. I told them that my family was in for the holiday and I could come in until after Christmas. I knew something had to be in the report because of the urgency in her voice.

We drove once again downtown to meet with the Neurosurgeon. I went to the appointment with the CD's from the Radiology department and the report. I was taken back quickly to the room and almost immediately the doctor flew into the room and asked me if I had seen the x-rays? I had not, I told him, he called me over to the computer so I could see.

It was a complete shock! I did not utter a single word. Clearly on the x-rays you could see where the lead wires for the stimulator were broken or fragmented as it was stated in the x-ray report. The lead wires were bent and two were broken away from the rest. I had no words.

The neurosurgeon let us know he has never seen this before. That it would need to be reported to the FDA. He was cautious in his approach; he did not know how to handle this. My husband and I were in complete shock. A thousand thoughts were circling in my head.

He ordered a 3-D CT scan next, he needed to see where the little fragment wire piece was. I did the CT scan quickly at my local hospital. We returned to get the results of the CT scan and he let myself and husband know that the results were not good. The piece of broken/fragment was sitting next to a major artery. That I could have a stroke or worse have an aneurysm. I had stayed strong throughout all of the things thrown out at me, infection, blood clots, clotting disorder, auto-immune disorders, amputation, and chronic pain. But I just couldn't stand strong now, I was being told that I could lose my life. I was going to lose my life because of trying not to be in unrelenting pain.

He let us know he would do what he could. Again, he told us that he had never seen this before and consulted with numerous neurosurgeons and none had seen this either. The neurosurgeon now scheduled me for an angiogram to find out if the piece was touching the artery or just next to it. I also needed to meet with his hematologist. He needed a team in the operating room and he wanted me to meet them all. I did as he asked, went to visit the hematologist first, pre-admission testing second and lastly the angiogram.

I met the neurosurgeon again, to get the results of the angiogram. Thankfully the results were ok, the piece was next to the artery but not touching it. We were able to schedule surgery. He has told me the risks of brain surgery and removal of the little piece of metal. He will remove the whole spinal cord stimulator and hunt down the little piece of metal with his team of surgeons.

My doctor's office informed me they scheduled my surgery for March 13, 2020. I was feeling anxious to have this ordeal over with, and I was feeling overwhelmed by the course of events. I have placed my trust and faith into this team of doctors to remove this metal fragment.

The coronavirus was just starting, but had not super emerged yet. I went to surgery, nervous, scared but ready to have the ordeal over with. The neurosurgeon met with us moments prior to surgery. Surgery went ok, I woke up in recovery with enormous pain. Finally getting that under control I went to my room. The nurse was asking me questions about myself and she wanted to see the incisions, I had three, one on my neck, one in the middle of my back and lastly where the battery pack was.

The nurse looked at the battery site and called another nurse in, she looked at it and called two other nurses in. Meanwhile I did not know, as I sat in bed what was going on. Since I had a history with infections, I thought for sure that is what was going on. None of the nurses would say a word. By now there were six nurses by my bedside and one without saying a word stuck a huge needle into my back. I had a Hematoma and she was trying to drain it. She was unsuccessful, I received an ace bandage and was told to keep it on.

I was discharged from the hospital; the fragment was found and my husband collected the SCS hardware from the Pathology department. I was happy to go home and start the recovery process. I was told that I needed to meet with several doctors since I just had surgery. One was the Hematologist. Since I have this clotting disorder, I needed to stop my blood thinners two days prior to surgery. I needed the okay from the Hematologist to go back on them. I met with him five days after surgery. He told me to wait until I see the Neurosurgeon before going back on the blood thinners. I remember looking at my husband who was in the room also and thinking ok, he is the specialist. Just a couple days later, I met with my general doctor. She inquired about the blood thinners and I told her what the Hematologist had told us. Shocked, she said, start the blood thinners.

Over the weekend, I was completely exhausted. I thought that I had just done too much. I slept for most of the day on Friday, Saturday and Sunday. I noticed it was getting difficult to breathe. The President had put the country in a quarantine, the news was flooded with the COVID 19 virus. I convinced myself I had the virus because I couldn't breathe.

On Monday morning, I took a shower and couldn't hold my head up. I knew something was wrong, but still convinced myself I had the coronavirus. My husband took me to the ER, because of the virus he was unable to come in with me. The ER asked me a ton of questions and ran a CT scan and ultrasound.

I did not have the coronavirus. I had a Deep Vein Thrombosis, Pulmonary Embolism and a collapsed lung. The hospital that I had surgery in the city, wanted me to be transferred to them. I declined and wanted to be close to my family. I left the ER and went to my hospital room. By now it was 9:00 pm in the evening. I was woken up by a Hematologist who came into my room and told me, if I stay here, I would die, if I go to the hospital in the city, you will live. And he walked out. Thoughts of my three boys and husband flashed in my thoughts vividly. The nurse came in and asked me what I was doing. Of course, I told them to transfer me.

I left in an ambulance to go to the hospital in the city. Each day I expected something special to happen, but I just received days of Heparin and then transitioned to Lovenox. They also ran heart tests, blood tests, CT scans and ultrasounds.

Still to this day I wonder why that Hematologist told me that. I think he was trying to hide the fact that the Hematologist I just saw days prior had told me not to take the blood thinners. That was a fateful choice, that I could have lost my life over. I was told if I would have waited to come in the outcome would have been different. I had clots in both lungs, a DVT in my left leg, the clot was so large in my right lung it had started to collapse my lung and started to cause heart issues.

For now, my journey still continues, I have CRPS not only in my hand but it has traveled to my right foot and now making its way to my left arm/hand. I do not know if it will continue to progress. I hope that I will be able to live a long and fulfilled life. My life will always include pain. I consider myself a person who tolerates a lot of pain and my pain level is high. Meaning I am able to handle a lot of pain before complaining. I have always said to many people, they wouldn't be able to sit inside my body for five minutes, but I live with the constant chain sawing.

CRPS is a pain that never turns off. I have over the years learned how to cope with it. It is unrelenting. It never stops. I try not to burden those around me with what I am going through. I try for the most part to be a very upbeat person, but oftentimes my days are filled with enormous pain. The kind of pain that makes you sweat, makes you cry, it completely encompasses my life. My outward appearance would never lead anyone to think I am dealing with this enormity.

I take opioid pain medicine, the kind that is in the news daily. Without this medication I wouldn't be able to function. CRPS has stolen many things from me, my sleep, my friendships, my sanity and my ability to even hold my husband's hand. I never thought that when I went to volunteer at a shelter, that I would leave with a lifetime of constant pain.

I do know after living with CRPS for numerous years, that most doctors do not have a clue the enormous amount of pain that CRPS causes. They don't have a clue that CRPS spreads and they do not have a clue on how to treat it. Many times, I am the one that is telling the doctors about CRPS.

I do not know if I could describe what it is like to have CRPS. But I do know often people say they experience a burning sensation. For me the best description it's like a chainsaw, but for those diagnosed with it, they are the strongest people in the world. To live a few moments with CRPS, is a feat, to live a lifetime in unbelievable pain is what heroes are made of.

WHEN A HUG HURTS
Claudette Johnston

In 1999, I fractured a triangular bone at the back of the ankle, called the Os Trigonum. I was 24-years old. In one week, I twisted my ankle on a stone in my driveway at home, and my heel got caught on new carpeting on the two-story stairs at work, days later. My heel got caught, and my foot lunged forward down two stairs. I was young and did not know I should have written an incident report.

I experienced pain that would only progress. Eventually, I consulted with a podiatrist who told me I had bone spurs. He placed me in a walking boot, and my ankle pain only continued to worsen. The doctor performed an injection for the pain, and it did not help. I started experiencing a sharp pulling pain that started in my ankle but went up into my leg. I had an MRI, which showed the fractured bone I mentioned previously. Unfortunately, I would require surgery. On April 19, 1999, my life changed in a way I never would have suspected. During the surgery, they discovered it to be a complex issue. I fractured a piece of bone that had lodged itself in my ankle joint, unbeknownst to my ankle surgeon. After my surgery, the cast was applied too tightly on my leg, and it caused damage to my sural nerve (sensory nerve), and the earliest version of the pain pump had caused an infection. They hospitalized me. I had cellulitis running up my leg. One of my specialists wanted to amputate. Thankfully, my primary doctor, Doctor C, rejected the idea. I was in the hospital for over two weeks. I had to be non-weight bearing for several months, and I had to relearn how to walk on my leg again.

I was fired from my job because I was too ill to return to work, and my doctor would not medically release me. He had diagnosed with CRPS, and eventually, referred me to the pain clinic, where my treatment journey began. I had so many different types of injections. I tried epidurals, trigger point injections, and Bier blocks, etc., but none of them were improving my incredible pain. The doctor at the pain clinic recommended I try a spinal cord stimulator (SCS) implant. To be honest, I was unreceptive to having the SCS. So, I naturally did some research, and I found a doctor from Florida who authored a book on CRPS. With the help of my parents, I went to Florida for two weeks of treatments with Doctor H.

We went to Vero Beach, Florida, which was a beautiful and warm place. We stayed at a hotel on the beach. Unfortunately, I wasn't able to walk on the sand. It was too difficult for me. I was there for two weeks of treatments with Doctor H. He recommended I should have a thermography test done to check for temperature irregularities in my extremities. It was from head to toe. The doctor diagnosed me with full-body CRPS. I had injections from the caudal of my spine to my forehead! It was terrifying and painful, but it improved my pain somewhat. I also had extremely swollen feet. I wore Teva sandals with Velcro so I could adjust the shoes according to my swelling. They gave me IV mannitol for edema and intravenous immunoglobulin (IVIG) for my depleted immune system. The doctor told my mom and me, I could've been close to death at home in the extreme frigid winter of Wisconsin. Cold is the enemy of CRPS! The doctor advised me to move to Vero Beach so I could continue with treatments five to six times a week. My life depended on it. And so, began my life's journey with CRPS.

Doctor H. would tell all of his patients not to overdo activity just because you had some pain relief and not to be too under-active. Both will only cause more pain. I could not live in Florida for more than a couple of months. I was too ill to live alone. I ended up in the ER a couple of times, and I had several treatments a week. Unfortunately, I began to have more health issues.

Over time, I have developed several other conditions, in addition to having CRPS. Currently, I suffer from diastolic heart failure, diabetes, high blood pressure, orthostatic hypotension, vasoconstriction, fibromyalgia, anxiety and depression, anemia, eosinophilic esophagitis, hypothyroidism, fatty liver disease, glaucoma, neuropathy and, several GI issues.

I have had many surgeries over the years. I've had two carpal tunnel surgeries, two ankle fractures, two back surgeries, and a hysterectomy, etc.

From the very beginning of my CRPS journey, my primary care physician, who has taken care of me, had mentioned several times that other doctors would not believe that I could be suffering from so many conditions. He knows that it is real, but feels that other doctors wouldn't believe it!

I have a question? Why are there so many doctors untrained in treating CRPS? My primary doctor informed me that CRPS goes away! The orthopedic doctor did not want to tell me I had CRPS. He only told me when I requested my records to consult with a different orthopedist. Finally, I met with a knowledgeable doctor who knew all about CRPS. He put me on proper medications and referred me to a pain clinic. I was not making up this unbelievable pain I was in. It was a real condition, and I could seek help for it!

Can you imagine having several different types of excruciating pain 24/7, without relief? It's unbearable! I have developed the following symptoms; crushing pain, zingers (electrical shocks), burning nerve pain, muscle spasms, and vasoconstriction are a few of my symptoms. With only the slightest touch to my skin, it sends pain waves throughout my body. Still, to this day, it hurts to wear socks! When someone hugs me, I feel pain. Imagine feeling so lost in illness and feeling left behind by most of my friends, whose lives were moving on. I was yearning for compassion, friendship, and a hug!! Having a chronic illness can be a lonely and solitary place, especially for young people.

Chronic pain can lead to isolation and loneliness. That's why it is important to hold tight to your family and friends. Seek support. You only need to ask! I know, wholeheartedly, that I couldn't have gotten this far in my journey without the unconditional love and support of my parents and friends. We lost my dad to health issues a few years ago. My mom is my rock and my best friend! I cannot imagine getting through 21-years of illness without her love and support. Due to some recent medical issues, that my mom is dealing with, our lives have turned upside down. She has been my caregiver and support system for many years. Now, I am taking care of my mom. It can be challenging and frightening at times. Please seek a support system. Talk with your family, friends, and don't be afraid to seek counseling. You should not feel less of a person, asking for help. I thank my family and friends for their support and love. My doctors have also been a great source of support too.

Please advocate for yourself! You deserve to be pain-free and to have your voice heard. Oh, and about those painful hugs, don't stop hugging me!!! I will gladly take a few minutes of pain for your loving gesture. Be well!! Sending you love and strength!!

THE INCREDIBLE CRPS JOURNEY
Lynda El-Mandouh

My Life Before CRPS

Before my injury, I was a normal healthy 41-year-old woman and a divorced parent for six years, with two young sons. I was an active person. I had bowled in leagues since I was 15-years-old, I enjoyed going on long bike rides with my sons, I did aerobic exercise every day, played tennis, was an active participant in both of my son's activities. I was the team's mother to the soccer kids and went to every practice and game. I also loved gardening, drawing, painting, refinishing furniture, and home improvement/remodeling projects.

I worked as an administrative supervisor for a major computer company, where I managed five people and traveled a lot for my work. I had a busy, fun life.

On July 13, 1986, I married my best friend, Mohamed; we were together for three years. He was my youngest son's soccer coach. For Mohamed, myself, and my children, life was full, active, and amazing.

Day of My Accident

September 6, 1990, started like any other day, up at 6:00 am to shower and get ready for work. Morning tea with my husband and sons, we talked about our plans and schedules for the day and evening, and I kissed everyone goodbye, dropped off my youngest son at school, and went on my way to work.

I had a conference call scheduled for that afternoon around 3:15 pm. My secretary had not given me the telephone number for a member of the out-of-state conference participants. So, I went back to my desk to retrieve the phone number and started to run back to the conference room. The next thing I knew, I was airborne! I landed on my right knee with my leg bent up underneath me.

At first, I hoped no one saw me fall. I felt so silly for falling. Then I tried to get up; the pain was excruciating, and I could not move. It must have been the only time in history that nobody was in that hallway. I laid there for what seemed like an eternity, but in reality, it was probably only a few minutes. Eventually, I could get up and limp back to the conference room. Both my knees were bleeding (my pantyhose did not get damaged—a great ad for L'eggs brand pantyhose), everyone (including me) had a wonderful laugh when I told them I had fallen. I left my office around 6:00 pm and could barely walk; both legs were stiff, but my right knee was so swollen, I could not bend or extend it.

I drove a five-speed shift and had a 40-minute drive to get home. I had to lift my right leg, by delicately holding my knee with both hands and moving my foot from the accelerator to the brake and back again, pushing down on my leg with my hands to speed up and slow down. I finally got home safely.

My right knee was now nearly four times its normal size; I placed an ice pack on it and took two aspirins. When Mohamed arrived home, he asked me what had happened? I told him I fell at work; he laughed at me and (so did I). Then, my sons arrived home; they asked me what happened to me? I told them, and we all laughed again. They all went off to soccer practice, and I stayed home to ice my knee and take another aspirin. They arrived back home around 9:00 pm, from their soccer practice, I was in so much pain, we decided I should go to the emergency room to have my knee examined and to find out what was causing all this pain I was having?

The hospital did X-rays, which confirmed that I fractured the patella on the right knee; and suspected I had soft tissue damage. I was informed to return the next day for further tests. Those tests revealed a torn meniscus cartilage and a fractured patella. They referred me to an orthopedic doctor who I saw a few days later, confirmed the diagnosis and suspected I had Reflex Sympathetic Dystrophy (RSD) (the new term for it now is complex regional pain syndrome (CRPS)) as my right leg (from the knee down) was now swollen, ice-cold, bluish-red in color, and felt as though it was on fire. The second opinion from both a neurologist and another orthopedic surgeon confirmed CRPS, and they gave me one page of information about CRPS.

The doctor determined surgery was necessary to repair the cartilage and patella, but he delayed the operation for a few weeks in an attempt to get the CRPS "under control." He placed my leg into a full length (thigh to ankle) wrap-around foam leg brace that had metal rods down each side, to immobilize my leg and a TENS unit attached to my leg inside the brace. I was only able to ambulate using a pair of underarm crutches.

My doctor referred me to a sports medicine rehabilitation clinic and received treatment four times a week. The treatment consisted of immersing my right leg into an iced whirlpool bath for 30-minutes, then I had to ride a stationary bicycle for 15-minutes. After that, the therapist would apply an ice pack to my right knee while they strapped it into a machine that would bend and straighten my leg out automatically every couple of minutes.

Pain, swelling, discoloration, and burning continued to increase, and my doctor finally scheduled my surgery for October 12, 1990. Fortunately, my surgeon was "somewhat" familiar with CRPS and elected to give me a spinal block during the invasive arthroscopic procedure, followed by a second block in the recovery room.

Life Immediately After an CRPS Diagnosis

At first, before the surgery, I had tried to go back to work (with the approval of my surgeon) two weeks after my accident. I still wore the full brace 24-hours a day and underarm crutches, I lasted one day at work.

I discovered one's inability to focus or function while in constant excruciating burning pain. I had already experienced the difficulty in trying to go to the bathroom at home, while strapped into a rigid full-length leg brace and on crutches. In the work environment, it was impossible in those small cubicles - I'll leave it up to the reader to envision that mental picture!

The work situation was further compounded by having a manager who was unsympathetic (pun intended) and who refused to make any allowances for my physical limitations, adjust my office hours or permit me to work from home. Therefore, my only option was to go home, and go on short-term medical leave and hoping I would recover with the surgery, ongoing physical therapy, and regular/daily pain medications.

I envisioned a return to work and getting my previous life back after a few weeks, (up to a few months), - right? I did not break anything - right? I still had both; my legs and there were many pain medications and therapies the doctors could prescribe - right?

At first, my new normal became regular visits to various doctors (several appointments each week), sports rehabilitation PT (twice a week), ganglion nerve blocks, done at the hospital, and a plethora of medications - too many to recount. I never felt comfortable taking opioids such as Morphine or Hydrocodone, that many chronic-pain sufferers' resort to, no judgment on my part, just my personal choice.

It also became apparent that "Sports Rehabilitation" PT was not appropriate or effective for CRPS. My doctor had now referred me to a Myofascial physical therapist, at first two-three times a week or as needed (PRN). It turns out that this PT method is more effective for my CRPS."

Life with CRPS

It became apparent, after about 18-months of frequent ganglion blocks and numerous different medications and doses, that none of these protocols/treatments were helping to reduce the pain; burning; swelling but instead caused major side effects and complications all of which exacerbated my pain and impacted me mentally, physically and emotionally.

I also developed an ulcer from being on NSAIDs for so long, so my doctor prescribed Cytotec to treat the ulcer. This problem caused severe vaginal hemorrhaging and caused me to lose nearly 30% of my blood 24-hours. I was very sick at this time. However, when my GYN doctor contacted Searle Pharmaceuticals, they informed her they have never heard of this side effect. Subsequently, it is an ingredient of the "morning-after pill."

By this time, I had begun to reluctantly consider the possibility that I might never go back to work, may never live without pain, continue to have ongoing complications from the "treatments," be in a wheelchair and or on crutches, or walking sticks for the rest of my life. Depression set in and overwhelming grief for losing "my life."

Also, by now I had gone from short-term disability (the first six months) to long-term disability, I battled for over a year with Social Security Disability (SSD) benefits, which my employer-mandated, I had to apply for after a year. I eventually won my case, and I accomplished this without a lawyer.

Also, I had become quite an expert in dealing with the dreaded Workers Compensation (WC) system! I thought SSD was a challenge, but once I won my case with SSD, I did not have to fight them any longer. It's not the case with WC; you have to fight them tooth and nail.

I had to fight the WC adjuster for everything. From the approval for medications, ongoing PT, adaptive equipment (crutches, walking sticks, electric scooter, etc.), and various doctor visits. These issues were directly related to my CRPS, but they were all consistently questioned and ultimately denied by the WC adjuster.

In the 1990s (and probably still today), the biggest battle was being believed and having to convince doctors, SSD, WC, employers, friends, family, and others that you are in this excruciating unexplainable pain after, a minor incident or injury and sometimes even the spontaneous development of CRPS.

My original injury was to my right knee, and there are undeniably visible symptoms that manifest with CRPS, and I had most of them. Here are just a few examples:

- Abnormal/accelerated hair growth: I had hair growing on the top of my toes.

- Abnormal nail growth and appearance: ridges and white spots in the nail.
- Discoloration of affected limb(s): purple, red blotchy skin. Shiny appearance. Feels as though it's on fire but is ice cold to the touch.

- Swelling of the affected limb(s).

- Excessive sweating caused by exacerbated pain levels, followed by nausea and dizziness.

- Physical reactions to cold, draughts, loud or a certain pitch of sound, bright lights and excessive heat (all of which severely exacerbated the symptoms of my CRPS).

Then there are the invisible symptoms, some but not all, that I experienced are as followed:

- Chronic sleep deprivation, even with sleep aides/medication I would only get three to four hours a night at most.

- Chronic short-term memory loss, my short-term memory was so affected that it was difficult to keep any recent information unless I wrote it down. I had to record all-important conversations to remember the details and appropriately respond. Before I had CRPS I never needed to write telephone numbers, I always had an excellent memory and could learn new procedures, names, and numbers with no problem. Now, I have to ask several times how to do simple tasks, which are embarrassing, tedious, and frustrating. I could be in the middle of a conversation with someone and suddenly lose all recollection of the topic or forget who I was talking too. On difficult days, I became almost ".panicked" if I had to make calls to unfamiliar people.

- Social interaction became almost non-existent. I could not make plans for social gatherings as I never knew what level my pain would be. I canceled many times, usually at the last minute, because my pain level prevented me from leaving the house. Some people eventually just stopped making arrangements with me.

- Chronic and severe constipation, the pain would double me over.

- I could no longer sweat except on the top of my lip and the back of my neck. Consequently, I was unable to tolerate weather with temperatures over 75 degrees, and I was at increased risk of heatstroke. The reverse was also an issue as I could no longer warm-up if I got cold. Temperatures below 60 degrees were a problem, hence during the summer month's air conditioning also caused me many issues.

The list could go on.

By the end of 1991, I had decided to stop all the medications except Zanaflex (which, in small doses provided some relief of the intense burning), ganglion nerve blocks, and anything remotely invasive or drug-related. I just continue with the Myofascial Physical Therapy, which had proven to give me some pain relief and had no side effects along with the Zanaflex.

At that time, doctors knew very little about CRPS. It seemed like every treatment was being thrown at me in the hopes something would work. Sadly, it did not help. The side effects, which only created more medical problems, which I then had to deal with, and it only further complicated my overall health and the ability to cope every day.

Suicide? I considered that "out," especially on those days, lying in bed curled up in a fetal position, in overwhelming pain, and unable to get up. When I could not put on clothes, cover with a blanket, or touch anything because of intense burning pain. Then I would think about the impact on my children, husband, mother, brother, other family members, or friends. To leave them feeling helpless, angry, and devastated that they could not "save" me. I have since seen what suicide does to a family, and friend's first hand, a dear friend of mine, a fellow CRPS sufferer took her own life, it was traumatic and devastating.

Do I blame her? No.

Do I miss her? Yes, every day.

Did I question whether I could have done more? Yes, absolutely.

I am just grateful I did not put my nearest and dearest through that awful distress and emotional pain.

I was fortunate to find a pain management specialist, Doctor D., who was not only supportive and open to my researching alternative treatments but also advocated on my behalf with WC and SSD. He was compassionate, understanding, and encouraging towards me. He would read all the articles and or publications I gave him and then discuss all the pros and cons with me. If I decided to try something, after doing my due diligence, he would back me 100% and compose "Letters of Medical necessity" when required. Unfortunately, Doctor D., eventually retired but referred me to his colleague Doctor James Cable.

Meantime, (between Doctor D., retiring and contacting Doctor James Cable) I saw several so-called "specialists" in pain management for CRPS - BIG MISTAKE!

One doctor I saw attempted to coerce me into having a spinal cord stimulator (SCS)implanted. Another tried to bully me into another knee surgery, and the physician's assistant of another doctor said: "you should be happy that at least you don't have cancer like Jackie Onassis."

Then, I remembered Doctor D's recommendation and called Doctor Cable, who was a clone of Doctor D, and has provided me with comprehensive and collaborative treatment and support for the last 22-years.

At the start of 1992, my dermatologist, who was treating the unexplained skin rashes and irritations that I would periodically have, told me about an article he read and thought I should do more research into it. This article documented the current research treating CRPS patients with Chinese acupuncture and electrical stimulation. This acupuncturist was Doctor Meng Sheng Lin, who was local to me. So, I decided reached out to her to make an appointment.

Although acupuncture can be invasive, with the use of needles. I wanted to see if it would help my pain. After a couple of preliminary meetings with Doctor Lin and the medical doctor, I decided to try this approach, after learning more about her research.

After having my first treatment, I achieved some relief from the pain and burning. Each subsequent treatment provided a little more pain relief. I was not pain-free by any means. I still had burning, swelling, and discoloration, but it was more tolerable and no adverse side effects from the treatment.

In February 1992, I continued the acupuncture treatments a few times a week (depending on my pain level) and continued with my PT sessions. Doctor Lin (Dallas Acupuncture Center, Richardson, TX) was my lifeline and gave me hope.

Around the same time, I discovered and joined a CRPS support group in my area run by a local physiologist, whose primary practice was focused on helping chronic pain patients. In 1993, the doctor had requested that I take over the support group. I told him that I would be more than happy to run the group.

Through working with our support group, I have met many amazing people and learned a lot from other support group leaders, patients from all around the globe, and the doctors who have been doing the recent research on this insidious disorder. Our support group has lost some CRPS patients, mainly through adverse reactions from procedures or medications, but we have pressed on.

I have received phone calls from CRPS patients located all over the world, and from patients diagnosed with Fibromyalgia. My telephone rang 24/7, and it was a little overwhelming in one way, but also surprisingly, comforting to know we were not alone, and yet the medical world still referred to CRPS as an orphan disease. In 1994, a group of doctors changed the name of this disease from reflex sympathetic dystrophy (RSD) to complex regional pain syndrome (CRPS) type 1 and 2.

Two landmark achievements of our small group were to participate in a satellite broadcast of the RSD conference hosted by the California RSDSA group on March 28th, 1998 and we also became a non-profit organization called " RSD/CRPS Association of North Texas" that same year.

In 1999, I decided it was time to resign from running the support group. It had been six years since I took over the group, and I was quite tired. Sadly, I could find no one to take over the group. At the end of that year, unfortunately, the group eventually folded until the psychologist who started the group, in the beginning, started it up again a year later. I believe?

During the preceding years, my CRPS had spread and was now "global" in my body. My CRPS began to spread from my right knee to the entire leg, and then to my left leg, left hand, face, chest, and right hand. Due to CRPS, I also suffered from osteoporosis.

The WC insurance company I was dealing with (through my employer's insurance) settled my case with me in 1996, agreeing to cover all related expenses for the treatment of my CRPS such as medication(s), PT, acupuncture and included any necessary adaptive equipment I needed: repair/replacement of wheelchair; an electric scooter; TENs unit; crutches/walking sticks, etc...

It was only in early 2000 that WC violated the agreement. They refused any treatments, adaptive equipment repair/replacement, PT sessions, and acupuncture. The insurance company defended its decisions by stating it was "not medically necessary." I tried to work with them directly, to no avail, so I had to file a bad faith case against them, and hired two lawyers who specialized in these types of cases.

In February 2000, my doctor diagnosed me with breast cancer. I was the fifth member of our support group of 59 members diagnosed with a different form of cancer. It was very frightening.

I had surgery in March and then six weeks of daily radiation treatments followed by a course of oral chemo and Tamoxifen. I could not tolerate this treatment and suffered side effects from it, so I stopped taking it after a few weeks. This issue happened to me while I was fighting with WC.

In December 2006 and January 2007, during this ongoing legal ordeal with WC, my PT clinic closed down, and my therapist referred me to Ms. Patti L. Schwartz from Centre of Physical Rehabilitation in Plano, TX (www.therapyatcpr.com). That is when my fight with CRPS took an upward path. At my first evaluation, Patti asked me if I had ever tried "cold laser therapy?" I told her I had never even heard of it.

Patti said that she had treated patients with CRPS before, but no one had this disease for as long as I experienced 17-years. I decided I had nothing to lose by trying cold laser therapy along with my PT.

I started my PT with Patti Schwartz in February 2007, which included the Myofascial PT complemented by the cold laser therapy. Bear in mind that up to this point in time, I was primarily ambulating in a wheelchair, on crutches, or walking sticks, and using an electric scooter.

At first, I started with a few PT treatments, plus the cold laser therapy a week, along with my ongoing acupuncture treatments. By September 2007, I was using my wheelchair less, except for bad days. Instead, I could get around with just using my crutches or walking sticks.

Now do not misunderstand me, there is no quick fix or magic pill in the treatment of CRPS. There were days when I had a difficult time getting into PT, screaming, and sobbing in pain. Living with CRPS is a lifelong journey, full of trial and error.

Slowly, but surely my chosen treatment protocol of regular Myofascial PT, acupuncture, and minimal medication was beginning to pay off. Gradually, my body and the CRPS adjusted to this routine.

In August 2007, I finally won and settled the bad faith case against WC. We negotiated an agreement to create a Medicare Set Aside (MSA) account. This account is funded by WC each year to cover my medical costs. They have this account managed through a third-party. Now, I never have to deal with WC or their representatives (adjusters) ever again.

I negotiated a clause that prohibits the MSA administrator the authority to "determine" whether (or not) any treatment protocol for my CRPS is medically necessary or if they will pay them at all. They must pay all bills received in full; no questions asked PERIOD! I also incorporated the annual annuity payment into the settlement agreement, and WC must pay it directly to me.

They also have to provide me with a lump sum of cash each year to pay for additional or miscellaneous expenses, not covered by Medicare, for the rest of my life.

I had been telling WC and their attorneys for seven years that I was not going anywhere. This fact was the rest of my life that I was fighting for, that I (not them) had to live with this insidious disorder, and the toll it had and would take on my body, general health, and quality of life. In my opinion, the outcome of this lawsuit would define me moving forward, for however long that would be. I believed that no matter what the result is, it must be in my best interest, not the results determined by WC and their lawyers.

Over the years, I lost count of the number of interrogatories, depositions, and affidavits I went through. I cannot remember how many "second opinion" doctors or clinicians WC sent me to. I believe all that was an attempt to (a) legally justify their denying any coverage for my CRPS, (b) hoping I would give up and go away, and (c) become too exhausted to continue the lawsuit. The dishonest behavior of WC, their attorneys, and their so-called doctors/clinicians only reinforces my resolve to continue. At the signing of this agreement, seven years after I initially filed it, the WC representatives and their attorneys audibly exhaled.

By 2008, I was ready to participate in something apart from dealing with my CRPS, doctor appointments, PT, etc... So, I decided to enroll in a Citizens Police Academy class offered by the local police department. They offered evening classes once-a-week for five weeks. I cannot describe the immense sense of achievement I felt when I graduated from the class. I took the next step and join the Citizens Police Academy Volunteers, a program where citizens help the local police in a variety of ways. The advantage of volunteering, apart from the satisfaction of being useful, and worthwhile, was its flexibility. The hours or days I "worked" were up to me, and on bad days I could stay home and on good days take part in an assortment of tasks and assignments.

It is now 2020, and I am still here, still having acupuncture, myofascial PT, along with cold laser therapy every week, and living my new normal. Do I still have CRPS symptoms: burning, swelling of hands, feet, legs, along with discoloration of limbs, and glossy skin. Yes! Is my pain still as debilitating? It can be at times. It does not flare up daily, as it used to, and apart from the significant odd sympathetic response (where I cannot function for a day or two), the benefits of this protocol, for me, have been remarkable. Life with CRPS can also be tolerable and manageable.

Over the past 30 years of living with CRPS, and discovering early on that if a product had "less than 2% risk of X, Y, and Z," I was that 2%.

I found a few products that provided relief without much risk of side effects (for me): Topical gels, creams, lotions - Feldene Gel, Equalizer Plus, and Deep Blue Cream. Electric Stimulation Therapy: gloves, socks, knee, or arm sleeves made from a soft woven conductive material, connected to a TENs unit, which sends a mild electrical current through the extremity.

I found that they can effectively reduce pain and swelling, especially flare attacks caused by changes in air pressure. All the items above are readily available online; when I first "discovered" some of these products had to be imported.

I believe the key for anyone living with a chronic illness, to be an informed patient; do your research; explore all your options; find a doctor that listens NOT dictates; a doctor that speaks with you NOT at you; reach out to others; join a support group. And last but not least, do not be afraid to ask for help.

There are still bad days, for me but there are also many good days too, I am enjoying life again.

THE NEVER-ENDING ROAD - CRPS
Robert Dutton

Let us go back to the starting line. My name is Bob, and I drove tractor trailers for 30-years and never injured myself. I retired from driving and went into sales. I was working at a high-end auto dealership and making a good living. One day, another salesperson came to my desk and said: "let's go have a smoke" I got up and off we went. On our way to the exit door, I slipped and fell down a flight of stairs and immediately knew something wasn't right. I was able to make my way outside but knew something was wrong. A few hours later, I was on my way home, taking off from work early.

The first stop was to my primary care doctor. He sent me for x-rays, nerve damage test, and finally an MRI of my lumbar spine. The doctor told me I had two discs in my lower back that had ruptured. He said I would probably need back surgery. My doctor then referred me to an orthopedic surgeon. I think you could guess what he was about to suggest to me. Yes, back surgery! Before having any surgery, I had to try pain medications, acupuncture, and chiropractic care. Of course, nothing helped me. So, in 2007, I went for my first of many back surgeries.

When I woke up from my back surgery, the surgeon told me he only repaired one level of my spine because when he looked at it with his naked eyes, he thought the second level looked good. I remember after the surgery; I had a terrible feeling about this situation. This issue was the beginning of my "opioid pain medication" affair. My problem was the pain never went away. Month after month, I would ask him, why am I still in pain? He would always give me the same answer, give it more time. Well, his time was up! I was frustrated, so I started looking for a new doctor.

During my research, I was shocked to find that the surgeon did not conduct proper tests to determine where my pain came from. Now, he is history!

My journey with complex regional pain syndrome (CRPS) begins. My wife made a phone call to a friend who had connections in the medical field and gave us the name of a new orthopedic surgeon. I remember sitting in the examining room thinking, here we go again. He recommended I have a discogram to find out where my pain was coming from. You guessed it again. It's from the area the first surgeon did not feel was needed to be repaired. I'm back on the operating table once again. This time, the surgeon had to remove all the hardware and start from scratch. I was on the operating table for 11-hours. After waking up, I remember thinking "what have I done." This time, I was in terrible pain. Any movement, or even blinking hurt. After surgery, I was continuing to ingest all kinds of pain medications, nerve medications, and muscle relaxants. This second surgery took place in 2008, and I was also diagnosed with CRPS. The pain never got better. I was given trigger point injections, facet joint nerve blocks, and nerve ablations, for which at the time they did not put you under, in fact, my doctor came in and gave me a towel to bite on and said: "this could hurt." Boy, was he right? I was screaming for him to stop but just kept hearing, "almost done."

Time moves so slowly when every day is the same, and you know you will be in terrible pain. From the minute you open your eyes until you try to sleep at night. I started doing my research on CRPS, and the information was all over the place. My back surgeon sent me to a CRPS specialist. At least, that is what he called himself. After giving me a hundred trigger point injections and still pumping opioids down my throat, I was still not feeling any better. Now, the pain specialist told me I need a spinal cord stimulator (SCS). He referred me to see a Neurosurgeon. This doctor said to me: "I will fix you right up." If that were true, then this would be the end of my story. Not even close to being true.

Spinal Cord Stimulator (SCS) #1. I spent nine days in the hospital while the doctor was trying to decide to make the SCS permanent or not. I received the trial version implanted first and remember waking up one morning to a nurse pulling on the leads connected to my spine. I said to her, "what the heck are you doing?" Those leads are attached to my spine." To make a long story short, they gave me the permanent SCS during a second surgery on the eighth day. I woke up and a representative from the company who makes the stimulator was giving me directions on how to use it but told me they would have to send me a new controller. That made little sense to me, but later I found out she had dropped the controller in the operating room, and my doctor refused to allow me to accept the original one. I wanted that equipment to work so badly. Now, my CRPS had traveled from my back, down my left leg and foot. The pain does not let up. When I take a shower, the water hitting my leg and foot almost sends me into tears. They implanted my first SCS in 2010. Now, they just give me more opioids, more injections, more of whatever they can think of to make money off of me. I have to travel monthly back and forth to the city just to get my prescriptions for pain. Did I mention this was a Workers Compensation (WC) case because I got hurt at work? Thus, anyone that has dealt with WC knows they fight you every step of the way. Every procedure and every surgery. Now, since there has been no evidence of improvement, my doctor decided I should now get a morphine pump, so he sent me to yet another doctor. This new doctor says I am a perfect candidate for a pump, but he cannot do it because he is in the middle of a new therapy drug trial for CRPS. He inquired if I would like to take part in the drug trial? I figured, what do I have to lose?

PRIALT.... the new wonder drug was going to resolve all my issues. Wait! I signed up to get injected with Snail Venom/Prialt. This treatment was merely supposed to be only a 15-minute procedure under live x-ray. Lying on my stomach, I felt the needle kept hitting my spine until I heard someone yell, "we have-a-leak." I yelled out, "what happened?" I got no response. After 90-minutes of being on the table, I was eventually helped up and directed to sit in a small recliner chair. I did not feel good at all, but after ten minutes, they informed me I could leave. No one instructed me of what was to follow. I should have laid down for a few hours before walking around to avoid getting terrible headaches. I made it home only to suffer a migraine for nine days. On the fourth day, I called the so-called doctor to determine what they could do, and he almost laughed, and said: "I could do a blood patch, but it might make things worse." So, I decided to deal with the headaches. His office called me a few weeks later and wanted me to have another round of Prialt, and double the dose this time. Now, it is was my turn to laugh. I was done with this Prialt treatment, as far as I was concerned.

The Pain: I do not know if I can describe the pain? The pain of CRPS is never-ending and worse than any pain I have ever felt in my lifetime. Your limbs swell up so much that you cannot even recognize your own body anymore, never mind your body changing different colors. I would take pictures when these changes happened, but the doctors never really cared to view them. One minute, your body can be on fire and the next, as if someone is stabbing you with a butcher's knife. Anyone who has this horrible disease knows that you will try anything to get just a little pain relief. So, that's what we do.

We try everything! Creams, ice, heat, pills, shots, and everything but the kitchen sink. One doctor wanted to give me Ketamine infusion treatments, but workers comp would not pay for it because they claimed it was only a

50/50 chance of success. Also, it sometimes only lasted for six months or so.

Next surgery: My orthopedic surgeon sent me for a CT scan of my lumbar spine, and it showed I have scar tissue pressing on a nerve, which was causing my pain. You guessed it, another back surgery. I go under the knife again, praying that this was it. Along the way, the doctor tells you: "this will fix it." Maybe some people are lucky? I was not lucky. After arriving home from a brief stay in the hospital, I could tell right away there was no change in my condition. Yes, there was nothing left to do, but go back to the medicine cabinet, to my old friend Oxycontin. I am now taking 80 mg of Oxycontin-ER every six hours along with 8 mg of Dilaudid every four hours, with 500 mg of Gabapentin every eight hours, plus Xanax and Baclofen. Whatever they told me to take, I took it, but I never exceeded the dosage. One time, I received a phone call from the workers' comp case nurse, informing me that if I continue taking my current medications at this current dose, I will end up in the ground. This time, I thought they just wanted to stop paying for my medications, since it was costing them around $60,000 a year just for my medications. It was something that had stayed in the back of my mind for a very long-time.

Spinal Cord Stimulator (SCS) #2: It's now 2016, and my SCS is not doing anything. So, my neurosurgeon told me they need to replace my SCS with a newer and improved model. For years, I have been chasing the proverbial carrot. I go back to the operating table again. This time instead of a nine-day stay, the doctor only kept me overnight. By this time, it seems like surgery is something you just get used to having. Something you expect you must do at some point. At the same time, you do expect some level of success. When that doesn't happen, it sends you into a deeper level of depression. More drugs. More shots. More procedures. This new

SCS works a little better than the first one did, but it still does not get the current down into my feet. I spent hours with the company's programmers that make the SCS, and we could not make the unit ease any of the pain in my feet. I now have a foot drop on my left side, which has caused me to fall down the staircase in my home (three times) from top to bottom. I have been very lucky at this point, not to have broken my neck.

Sleep is a luxury for very few patients with this disease. The only way to get some sleep is to over-medicate yourself. I have tried every over-the-counter pain medication, so maybe it's time for a different plan of action? Maybe, I should try "medical marijuana?" I have heard that it could help me sleep at night? So, now it's time to find yet another new doctor so, I can get registered with the state of New York, where it is now legal to use medical marijuana for chronic pain and other medical conditions.

Medical Marijuana: After searching and searching, I found a doctor in NYC that could help me get my certificate to register for medical marijuana. My first office visit, he hands me paperwork to fill out, then his "girl Friday" put her hand out and says "that will be $300.00 please." I assumed that was it. I got home and after reading my new certificate I noticed it expired in 30-days. WHAT! I make another appointment, and when speaking to this doctor, he told me the State only allows him to give me a certificate for 30-days at a time. There goes another $300.00! This issue has been going for six months. One day, while I was at the dispensary, I was talking with the pharmacist and told her what my doctor was charging me, she then slipped me a note like in a James Bond movie that had the name of a nurse who could give me a certificate good for one year at a time for only $200.00 a year. I was happy and mad at the same time. I now try to pass her information on to anyone I can, to help save them money. I took WC to court trying to get them to pay for my medical marijuana using an MG2 form, but I got a judge who was not having it. He acted as if I belonged in jail. It now costs me between $300.00 and $500.00 per month to buy my pain medication that WC should pay for. So far, medical marijuana is the best pain treatment I have tried so far. I am told that you need to have some level of THC for the CBD molecules to piggyback-ride to the correct pain receptors in your brain, or it is a waste of time and money. I use a 50/50 blend of THC and CBD. Now, at first, it made me a little high, which I wasn't happy about, but after my body adjusted to it, I was fine. I am still taking all my prescribed medications from my doctor, and use medical marijuana for breakthrough pain, and to help me sleep.

Dropped like a hot potato, I had been treating with the same pain management doctor for 12-years. Then, suddenly with no notice, at my next office visit, he tells me goodbye. I said what! He is no longer accepting WC for payment from this point onwards. Now, put yourself in my situation. I am taking high-levels of medications and this so-called "crisis" is not helping my case. I told him; I can never find another physician who will give me what I take now as a new patient. He did not care. I was frantic now! After a few days of searching, I found a new doctor who was willing to help me as long as I promised to lower my intake of medication. I had no idea what I was agreeing to. In one year, I was able, with the aid of medical marijuana, to lower my medications to 15 mg of OxyContin ER three times a day. I also stopped taking Dilaudid completely. No more Xanax although, I take a 5 mg Ativan once in a while if I am experiencing a bad day. I also lowered my Gabapentin to 300 mg three times a day. The problem with all this is that my pain levels are through the roof, and there's no going back.

The road traveled to lower my medications was not a pleasant one at all. I was sick all the time, and it increased my pain. I guess it's all worth it?

I am in the same boat again … now Covid-19 hits. It hits New York hard. People are afraid to leave their homes. This added stress is making my pain soar. Then comes another blow, my pain doctor is leaving her current practice, and where she is going, she can no longer prescribe opioids. I simply cannot win for trying. I am back on the search again for a new doctor. I have talked to doctors about the new DRG stimulators for which they tell me…. wait…you guessed it; it can fix you, Bob! It seems like I have heard this before. The number of doctors willing to hand-out opioid medication for any reason has gotten almost non-existent. After all the treatments and procedures, I have been through, I am not looking to start over with a new doctor and, "I can fix you." I have an appointment at a new practice middle of June. I am nervous about Covid-19 and not sure what my future is. Not a good place to be at this time.

My final thoughts: CRPS is a disease that takes everything away from you. It takes your body, your mind, your friends, and your family. You can never make advanced plans. Sometimes you can go somewhere with your friends, and 20-minutes later, you are in pain and want to go home. You go through different stages. I think anger is the worst one to get loose from. It had a hold on me for a long time. You ask, Why me? What did I ever do? Many things cause it. A simple twisted ankle, a sprained finger, it's so unpredictable. No cure! They do not teach doctors about this disease in medical school, which is wrong. At least that's what I have been told by many upcoming doctors. I thought I was too young when I developed this disease at 54-years-young. After 13-years of dealing with chronic pain, my heart goes out to the younger people who have to suffer their entire life. At least, I got to live more than most have. Please do your research, ask questions, do not keep trying to reach for the proverbial carrot. Below is a list of procedures and medications that I can remember having and taking.

Procedures:
Ablation of nerve endings from L3-S1
Faucet Blocks at L4-S1
Trigger Point injections – at least 100
Acupuncture
Chiropractic Care
Two spinal cord stimulators
Total of seven failed back surgeries - fusion L4-S1

Medications:
Oxycontin
Oxycodone
Morphine
Baclofen
Amitriptyline
Gabapentin
Prialt
Xanax and Ativan
Medical Marijuana

At this point, this is all I can remember. Things start to fade after being in such terrible pain for so many years. CRPS is the hardest thing I have ever had to deal with and wouldn't wish this on anyone. Good Luck, Everyone.

One last thing. This disease has taken all the fun out of my life. I fight each day not to give in to depression. I have lost all my friends and understand why. People want to make plans with you and you want that also, but you are torn. You get a call, let's go to dinner next Thursday.
You want to say yes, every bone in your body wants to go, but your automatic response is to say no. You are afraid that if you say yes, then either you will have to cancel at the last minute or you will make it to the

restaurant, and halfway through the meal, you have to leave. So, you do not spoil everyone's time, you just say no to everything. After you keep disappointing your friends and family, slowly over time, they just stop asking you. Very few people understand the mental battles we deal with daily. Pills don't stop your mind from thinking, would have, could have, should have. It's very difficult not to give in to anger or a sense of worthlessness. You may start as the life of the party, always with the jokes. Life has a funny way of playing jokes on all of us, except I am not laughing anymore.

I wonder what would my life would have been like if I had not developed this disease CRPS? I used to snow ski, even offered a job as a ski instructor at Mt Snow Resort in Vermont, I was much younger back then, but I still loved to ski. I used to be on a bowling team and did well with a 188 average. Now, I cannot even lift a bowling ball, much less throw it down an alley. My trucking company had a softball team for which I played shortstop every weekend. Now, I cannot even sit long enough to watch a game, much less take part. I think the worst physical damage, on top of the disease, would be that the lack of mobility has caused my body to load itself up with arthritis. A few months ago, I had to have a complete shoulder replacement surgery for which I believe was because of always walking with a walker and the lack of movement. I also believe that my long-term opioid use has damaged some of my organs. Most days, I am in too much pain to do anything at all, but I still try to play my guitars. That's my therapy!

A brief note. Trying to describe the pain would be futile, but I can tell you that three times I asked my orthopedic surgeon to amputate my left leg. That was before the disease progressed into my right leg. He declined but said if he thought it would end my pain, he would do it. He explained that the phantom pain after losing my leg could be worse. So happy not to hear "that will fix it."

My wife is an Ovarian Cancer Survivor and depends on me to be there for her to continue. We have a beautiful 4-legged daughter who depends on us for everything. If not for that, I would probably have given up years ago. Maybe?

There are thousands of conditions that cause chronic pain, but we all share the day-to-day struggle of just making it to tomorrow. Some will not make it to see tomorrow's sunrise. This is just my story, my opinions, you must try to be strong.

Take chances, find a good doctor, and put your trust in them. If you can, try to make chronic pain a term from the past. Fight for your children and future grandbabies, so they do not have to suffer as we did!

I am currently waiting to hear back from my local Congressman as I have requested a meeting to discuss some state law changes. Wish me luck! Let's all try to make a difference.

Thank you very much for reading about my life. Please do not make the mistake of neglecting your health. Once you enter the never-ending road, there is no end! Good luck and be well!

Robert Dutton
Brooklyn, New York

THE FOURTH OF JULY- CRPS WITH A BANG!
Laura Anderson

My complex regional pain syndrome (CRPS) story started on July 4th, 2018, when I fell going down some steps. They rushed to our local emergency room by ambulance. While in the emergency room, the doctor diagnosed me with a pilon fracture of my tibia and fibula at the thickest part just above my left ankle. The doctor tried to align my bones, but he could not do it, so he put a splint on my leg, gave me some pain pills, a pair of crutches, then sent me home with a list of orthopedists to call.

I saw an orthopedist doctor two days later, and he decided to admit to the hospital that day. Because of two days of swelling made a corrective procedure impossible, the surgeon could only attach an external fixator to my injured leg. He said that despite my broken bones, I had not compromised the ankle joint.

Ten days later, I was hospitalized again for surgery to repair my broken bones. The six-hour procedure included three titanium plates and thirty screws above my left ankle.

I knew I was in trouble when I woke up after my second surgery. My foot became swollen beyond recognition, and the pain was beyond anything I've experienced before. I was not on an orthopedic floor because they had no beds available. I had to request that the head of pain management for the hospital come to see me after five hours of crying in pain. She helped me get things under control. I was in the hospital for about five nights.

I spent the next six months doing PT three times a week and once a week in aqua therapy. I worked with acupuncture, pain management, and my trainer when I could push through the pain.

They told me my symptoms resulted from CRPS. Despite all of my hard work, including various devices, to stretch my foot, manual massage, stretching, etc. I could not get my foot past neutral flexion.

I was fortunate I was able to get an appointment with a leading foot and ankle reconstruction surgeon for a second opinion. He immediately saw that they had screwed my ankle in the equinus position during the corrective surgery.

In September 2019, the second surgeon lengthened my Achilles tendon and removed one plate, but was unable to increase the ankle flexion. My foot is deformed now, but I can walk with a cane and can stand for a few seconds unassisted on my injured leg. I continue to work out virtually with my trainer, ride my elliptical, and can walk about a mile sometimes.

I have soft tissue damage and neuropathy in my impacted limb. I tried Ketamine, and it was tremendously helpful, but I am having bladder problems now so, I am not sure if that will continue to be an option. I will resume swimming laps as soon as the pools reopening.

Thank you, for reading my story.

Laura

COUNT YOUR BLESSINGS INSTEAD OF PAIN
Ann S.

CRPS January 2000

Right Knee replacement surgery! The day was finally arriving – January 8, 2000. After six months of being on crutches and in immense pain, I was going to get the problem taken care of and get rid of the horrible pain. All I was wanting was to be able to dance with my husband again, play on the floor with my grandchildren, walk without crutches, and play with my fur babies. I thought I could manage the pain from surgery and recuperating to reach these goals. Plus, I would be back to work in a few months.

On the day of surgery, my youngest son gave me a note with the following scripture written on it "**Isaiah 40:31** – "But they, that wait upon the LORD shall renew (their) strength; they shall mount up with wings as eagles; they shall run, and not be weary; (and) they shall walk, and not faint" Little did I know just how much this scripture would come to mean to me over the next 20- plus years.

I knew immediately after having my surgery that something was not right. I could not stand having the bedsheets to touch my right knee area. Taking strong pain medicines did not help my pain. I just could not sleep, my knee and leg burned like a bad sunburn and it itched constantly. They gave me no explanation at the hospital why this was happening? After almost three weeks in the hospital, I came home, and the pain and sensitivity only got worse. We had an enclosed hot tub, and I would get into it but had to turn the jets off because they hurt my knee and leg. The only way I could sleep was to place my head on a towel as I sat in the hot tub with the warm water on me. To help me go to bed at night and try to sleep, my husband built me a "cage" apparatus so it would keep the covers from touching my knee and leg. I could no longer wear long pants, skirts, or jeans (I still cannot wear them after 20-years).

This started my six weeks of research, depression, and persistent pain. Finally, I had an appointment with the doctor who did my surgery. It was then he told me he thought I had complex regional pain syndrome (CRPS). Hallelujah, I had a name for what was wrong. It was not all in my head like my family members were saying. I was not crazy. My husband and I came home and immediately looked up CRPS on the internet. After reading about it and realizing that there was not a cure for it, I went into a deeper depression.

I started my endless rounds of going to doctors and pain specialists. Everybody seemed to have unique ideas on causes, treatments, etc. They all said there is no cure for CRPS. I had a series of nerve blocks but had no relief from any of them. I tried a TENS unit, went to psychologists to help handle the pain and depression, more opioids – stronger opioids. With the original pain, I had lost 25 pounds, and I called it the "pain diet." Taking the medications, I soon gained over 40 pounds. The "powers in charge" started talking about surgery to help me. I had read enough by then to know that I did not want surgery and have the disease spread. So, I gave up!

My husband told me to go online and find a doctor somewhere in the United States that could help me. Looking for this "miracle doctor" led me to a Mr. Eric Phillips, who told me about Doctor Hooshmand in Florida. Eric explained that Doctor Hooshmand stayed booked up, and it might be a while before he could see me. So, I called him anyway. Doctor Hooshmand had me booked for an appointment within a few weeks.

It was with a lot of prayers and faith, along with fear and trepidation that we went to Florida. On the first day, I met Doctor Hooshmand I knew he was my answer. It was through his caring, his advice, and his treatments that my pain became livable. Doctor Hooshmand never promised me a life without pain or a miracle cure or treatment. He promised me he would help me and would guide me so that my CRPS would not get unlivable. I will say that it alarmed my husband when he saw the shots the doctor would give me because of the size of the needles and how he gave them to me. He would sit in front of me and hold my hands, and I could always tell when Doctor Hooshmand was about to give me a shot because my husband's eyes would be as big as saucers. The doctor and his nurses quickly learned that I would start holding my breath and would not breathe regularly, and I can still hear them say to me, "Breathe Ann, breathe!"

I had to quit my job as an administrative assistant and, like many others with chronic diseases, became financially strapped. We were going to Florida about every four months. On one of the trips, Doctor Hooshmand wanted to do a Thermography (infrared thermal imaging) on me, but my insurance would not pay for it. I think it was going to cost us around $300.00? So, I had to tell Doctor Hooshmand that we could not do it. He got angry and said he would pay for it himself. The Thermography showed the "fire and ice" of the disease called CRPS. Taking non-addictive pain medicines, and taking warm Epsom Salt baths became a way of life for me. Trying to get more rest was a part of what Doctor Hooshmand wanted for me. He said, "To fight pain you have to have rest because it takes so much energy to fight the pain." How true a statement that was?

I was traveling alone to my appointment with Doctor Hooshmand, and read me a riot act, and told me never to do that again. He and Eric made sure that I returned to my hotel safely after treatment, and under their care, I felt safer. Having caring people around you, especially your doctors and nurses, it makes a world of difference. If you do not have that, then you need to find someone else.

When Doctor Hooshmand retired, it broke my heart. We went back to Florida a few times, but then we stopped going. I decided that I would handle my CRPS on my own. My primary care doctor said he would prescribe the pain medicines that I needed. At that time, I was taking only one medication, as I had gotten off all the addictive medications. Now, I only use one medicine, and I do not take sleeping pills because they do not work for me.

Thankfully, the CRPS stayed just in my right leg for the next five to eight years. There were side effects and precautions I had to take. Doctor Hooshmand warned me about things not to have done. Blood started showing up in my urine, nothing you could see except by a microscope. It was never an infection but came from the CRPS. I started having problems with my teeth, and I knew I should not have a root canal as that trauma was a greater risk than being put to sleep and having the tooth removed. I knew the dentist had to give me two to three times as much medicine to deaden my mouth as he would a "normal" patient and explained that to him before I consented to be his patient. I also wanted him to have the option to say he did not want to treat me due to the CRPS. Always let every doctor you go to know that you have this disease and what can and cannot be done to you. Also, explain the risks once you know the risks. I always lived in fear that I would get hurt and the disease would spread but knew that I couldn't live in fear, but would just have to trust in God more to keep me safe. A portion of my back also became very sensitive, and I have to be careful of that. Later my right foot started hurting, burning, and freezing at the same time. One of the weirdest things was my internal body thermometer was getting more and more unreliable. Anything over 75 degrees and I would easily get overheated and sick. Many times, I have barely made it back into my house and, without taking off my clothes, get into a cool shower to cool myself down quickly. You learn how to handle whatever this disease throws at you. You have to!

You must have a sense of humor through trials, and you need a sense of forgiveness in others and yourself. One example that I am not proud of is this one. The painful flare-up had gone on for days, and we had to cancel plans to meet friends for dinner. I somehow got onto the floor and started hitting my CRPS leg and cursing God out for allowing me to have this disease. Believe me, when I say God forgave me a lot quicker than I forgave myself. I can say I have never done that again.

Six years ago, I started having problems with my left eye. The vision was getting worse, but the doctors could not find out why. We concluded that the CRPS was the culprit. I was talking to specialists for months and months; we made the decision that I needed a cornea transplant, but the greater risk of the CRPS spreading to my face outweighed the surgery. I know that one day I may not see out of that eye, so I am trying to take measures in using it now such, as using a Kindle with a light on it, where I can control the font size as needed. I had to have laser surgery on that eye, and the doctor had deadened it and started the surgery. I almost jumped out of the chair and yelled. He asked me what was wrong, and I told him he hurt me. He did not believe me at first and started again. Again, I yelled. He asked me if I could stand a few more seconds of the pain as he was almost finished. So, a nurse held me still while he finished the procedure.

He was amazed. He told my son (who is an optometrist) that he had done this surgery thousands of times and never had a patient say it hurt them. He knew I was not faking it as it caused my heart rate to speed up and my

BP to go astronomical. He sent me straight across the street to the emergency room at the hospital.

Two years ago, I woke up one morning and could bend all my fingers into a tight fist. By that evening, I could not bend my middle finger on my left hand. A week later, I could not bend my ring finger and two weeks later I could not bend my little finger. I do not have arthritis. I had an MRI done on my hand, and the diagnosis revealed the CRPS had moved into those three fingers. After a year of physical therapy, I still could not bend or use them. Two years later, those three fingers are still misshapen and discolored and are not usable. My husband has to cut my food for me. I cannot peel vegetables anymore, and he helps me make the bed and change the sheets. Thankfully, I am right-handed or this could have been much worse for me.

Over the years, the name of the disease had changed from reflex sympathetic dystrophy (RSD) to complex regional pain syndrome (CRPS). A NEW NAME – THE SAME PAIN. No matter whether you call it RSD or CRPS, there is still no cure and no designated treatments. Many doctors and nurses still do not know about this disease even though it is listed on pain charts as one of the most painful. It is not genetic which is one of the only good things about it. It is not a visible disease so others cannot see it and think you are okay. It is not a known disease where people know someone about it and can understand. This disease can put enormous strains on marriage, and at times on my sanity. My husband and I have had some testy moments and rough months, but I am one of the blessed ones in that he has stayed with me and helped me and loved me through (or despite having) CRPS. I have lost some friends who just never could understand how I needed to break an appointment with them at the last minute because I never got to sleep the past couple of nights or the rain has made it worse or stress has made me flare-up. I have also made new friends — friends that both have the disease and others that do not but are just put here to bless me.

I was 55-years-old when I had my first right knee replacement surgery. Ten years later, at age 65, I had to have another knee replacement surgery again because the first one broke apart. Yes, this second surgery was something that I had to have done. I knew it could make my disease worse, and it did, even with taking all the precautions before, during, and after the surgery. I am now 76 years old, and I have worn a brace on my left knee for 17-years because I need surgery on that leg too, but I will not take the risks. I use an electric scooter when we go away from my house, and I can go camping with my husband. I cannot work in my yard as I used to love to do, but I can sit on my front porch with my little dog and watch my husband take care of things. I still cannot dance with my husband, but our love is greater now than ever before. I cannot walk on the beach or swim in the ocean, but I can take my scooter on the pier and go fishing. I do not drive anymore, but I can still stay in touch with my friends through Facebook, emails, and phone calls.

Through the years, I have learned to live by this motto, "Any day you can count more blessings than pain is, indeed, a gift from God." Sure, some days I may have to thank God for even the blessings of the smallest things, but I always seem to have more blessings, which gets me to the next day.

That scripture-verse that my son gave to me before having my first surgery and getting my diagnosis of CRPS. It is still my favorite. I know that one day that eagle will be me as I run and not grow weary, and walk and not grow faint, and I WILL soar like an eagle, and I will not hurt anymore.

THE DIAGNOSIS NO ONE WANTS
Traci Lundy

My story starts on Thanksgiving Day 2013, at the Honolulu International Airport baggage claim carousel, where I rushed to claim my 50-pound suitcase. I was wearing platform slides that broke when the suitcase hit my right ankle. My foot inverted when hit then reversed as I tried to straighten my foot. I hurt myself! Not realizing my shoe was broken, I walked painfully to the taxi pickup. During the taxi ride, I examined my injury.

No wonder it hurt so much to walk. The platform on my right foot had no strap inside to hold the shoe on my foot. It was very embarrassing! Vacation began at the military resort Hale Koa. Shoe shopping would be my first stop. The resort was amazing. Something was so weird with my foot, and I also noticed that both of my feet looked swollen, red, and way more painful than it should be. I took pictures with my phone and emailed the story home to my family. No problem-I knew about RICE (Rest, Ice, Compression, and Elevation) after injury. You can relieve pain and swelling and promote healing with RICE. Admittedly, this treatment did not help as much as it should have, but why did both feet look the same? I pushed through the pain with a few massages and considered an appointment with a doctor, but what could they do for me? The pain was awful, but I had seen much worse sprains. I constantly explained to myself and others, "I hurt myself and cannot walk well." I apologized for myself and planned to go see Doctor F., my family physician when I returned home. It was so crazy! I even broke a brand-new pair of flip-flops. The flight home was so unbearable I cried.

It has been over six years since I read the letters "CRPS" in my patient record. In my twenty-five years of working as a registered and licensed

Dietitian. I had reviewed many patient charts but skimmed over the "possible CRPS" I did not even recognize it as a potential diagnosis.

Treatment Timeline

December 2013: Doctor F., did X-rays with no findings, gave me a steroid injection, and prescribed Voltaren topical gel. By the end of the month, the asymmetrical rash was present on both shins. The swelling and pain were unresolved and worsening.

January 2014: I discontinued Voltaren and returned to Doctor F., where he taped my right foot. This is the most relief I have experienced since returning to full-time work after vacation. They referred me for a podiatrist appointment the following week. The pain and swelling were getting worse, so the doctor repeated the X-rays. Doctor N., did not understand why I was crying as he tried to fit a short walking boot on my foot. It hurt! No way would I take the walking boot for a suspected diagnosis of Plantar Fasciitis. Doctor N., was mad or upset, too. He told me he had nothing else to offer unless I would undergo an MRI.

The MRI hurt worse than the walking boot, and I felt like it would never end. Walking throughout the hospital was excruciatingly painful. The MRI results showed a torn ligament and tendon damage. I agree to the walking boot and receive a steroid injection in my foot. The "rash" is angrier now with sores of some kind. I said this is not going to help. I call an orthopedic foot specialist Doctor D., for an evaluation. I don't know how much longer I can work a demanding job with travel required when I can barely walk or drive?

February 2014: Doctor D., could not touch or examine my foot without me crying. I left his office with a cast up to the knee, and a recovery estimate of four months. I do not know how I can wear business clothing, so Doctor

D., writes a note for my work, and I apply for intermittent FMLA. I want to continue working, but this workplace environment is not supportive. After 25-years of service, it is time to retire later this year, 2014. I am certain a new work- environment will be a much-needed change for me.

March 6, 2014: After a month of being driven back and forth to work by my husband, I get my cast off my and get a new tall walking boot. My symptoms return with a vengeance.

April 2, 2014: I get a second casting. Another month and my husband must drive me to work. I do not understand why I cannot get a diagnosis? I am not making this swelling, redness, and pain up.

May 2014: Doctor D., told me there was nothing left he could do for me and was referring me to pain management. I did not understand? Something was wrong! I get my medical records, walk out on crutches, and try a pain management clinic. I did not know what to expect from pain management, but they treated me like a criminal. All I want is help but, seriously, I will not accept a $1,000.00 foot cream after being accused of "opioid seeking." In my defense, I had "pain pills" at home and never took them.

I call a different orthopedic, Doctor M., who was highly recommended to me by a colleague. He took X-rays, looks at my MRI, reviewed Doctor D's., notes, and did an exam (mostly range of motion), and told me Doctor D., had suspected "CRPS" and he agrees. This diagnosis requires Lyrica and a lumbar sympathetic nerve block followed by physical therapy.

My Anesthesiologist, Doctor RD., was so kind. He asked if I knew the procedure and why I was doing it? Well, no, I understood this was my path to recovery. He explained to me, something I heard for the first time, this is **"The Diagnosis No One Wants."** My first lumbar sympathetic nerve block offered so much pain relief that I was hopeful!

June, July, August 2014: Six lumbar sympathetic nerve blocks followed by physical therapy (during my lunch hour) three a week. I was finally getting better, but six was the maximum number of blocks. What then? I started researching CRPS and possible experts. During these three months, I was drawn to a local "CRPS expert," Doctor JM. He wanted me to discontinue my care with Doctor M., and Doctor RD., and continue Lyrica and physical therapy and add a pricey foot cream with Ketamine. If my symptoms were unresolved in two years, he would offer me a spinal cord ablation and/or a spinal cord stimulator (SCS). After one very painful nerve block, I knew I had made a mistake and had to ask Doctor R.D., to PLEASE me fix my mistake. I had no experience with how different the same procedure can be with another doctor.

September, October, November, December 2014: I went to see Doctor K., (in Tampa, Florida) who has a vast knowledge of CRPS, and intravenous Ketamine infusions. I had the best evaluation, treatment, information, recommendations, and hope yet. When I left, I could finally taper off Lyrica for good and start warm water exercise. I knew I was one of the lucky ones because I had no pain or swelling! I retired from my career a year after my injury. I would find my dream job. Also, I was in debt because I took a second mortgage to pay for CRPS medical treatment.

January 2015: The cold-winter has been unkind. Although the warm water exercise has given me help; I cannot concentrate, do simple personal health care, house duties, wear shoes, or most of my clothes.

The pain and swelling have now returned. Hot water and Epsom salt foot soaks are helpful for swelling and pain. I did apply for SSDI with my husband's help.

February 2015: My attitude and despair have caused me to retreat inside myself. I cannot do anything so, what good am I? I am very unhappy and do not want anyone to see me this way. It upset my husband, and rightfully so. Unfortunately, he has his first LAD heart attack. So, I must step up to this challenge somehow!

March, April, May, June 2015: I continue warm water exercise to the present day, even teaching a water class to people with Multiple Sclerosis, Arthritis, and others with painful conditions. My primary care, Doctor F., helps me start Low Dose Naltrexone (LDN).

My SSDI is approved. I bought a manual wheelchair and still wish for a SmartDrive wheelchair with power assist someday, but (Insurance and/or Medicare will not help with most treatment and mobility devices for CRPS).

My husband and I travel to Arkansas for a chance at the Neridronate Clinical Trial. It is a double-blind study with two different doses. Neither dose is the full 400 mg dose provided in Italy, and I am not accepted to participate.

The search for an I.V. Ketamine Clinic has begun. The obstacles are many. My husband had a fall down the steps in our two-story home. I cannot even make it up the stairs to sleep most nights and use a heating throw on my legs for relief even to the present time. We are selling our home and moving to a one-story, disability-friendly home.

July, August, September, November, December 2015: Fortunately, I had found the perfect person to hire for helping us with moving our home. I move so slowly; that without her help, I could not have managed this enormous task. I found a pain management doctor in town, providing Ketamine infusions. I was excited about this opportunity and becoming a patient of Doctor N.

January, February, March 2016: The winter-cold is back! The opportunity with Doctor N., just never materializes for many reasons. The bottom line, he could not provide the I.V. Ketamine infusions. During my continuing research for a CRPS Ketamine clinic, I discover the President of Mountain View Clinical Research, Inc., Kristen Johnson, BS, RRT, CCRC. We meet for lunch to discuss a new Ketamine Clinic in Denver, Colorado. I will be their first low-dose Ketamine patient.

April, May, June 2016: I booked travel and lodging for the two weeks' "loading dose." My husband drove to Denver, and I took the one-hour flight because long-travel is not possible for me anymore.

Doctor JK., is an experienced CRPS pain medicine specialist. He and Kristen provided compassionate care and treatment. My pain and swelling disappear again during the Ketamine infusions, but I must return every three months for a three-day booster. I continue this treatment regime to the present day.

January 2017 through January 2018: I started the Neridronate full dose, clinical trial participation with Kristen and Doctor JK., was full of high expectations. In reality, I achieved reasonable relief in a timeline different from the pharmaceutical company's research model.

February 2018: My husband had his second heart attack. So very frightening. He handles everything well. I'm so proud of him. My caregiver doesn't quit. He works, exercises, cooks, cleans, does laundry, grocery shops, and runs a whole lot of errands. He has so much to give to me, family, friends, and others. He is an inspiration!

Conclusion: There is still a lot to learn and many things I will never understand. I have CRPS in both legs and feet. I've never experienced "remission." I don't relate to some CRPS Community terms, for example, I would never describe myself as a Spoonie, Warrior, or Survivor. I do think of myself as disabled. Disability is not something a person chooses but "it is what it is." Admittedly, I spend time wishing it were different because I miss so much: going for a walk, riding a bike, dinners out, Sunday church service, and working. I am mostly home bound and want to be a more active wife, mother, grandparent, daughter, sister, and friend.

My feeling is that aging plays a role in my treatment as the CRPS progresses I have thought about how I should deal with increased mobility problems and I have been on a waiting list for a service dog (available to Military Veterans) for several years. I'm not sure if it is in my destiny?

I know, for certain, that I have learned to be grateful for what I have. Maybe that's my biggest lesson of all! Gratefulness helps me focus on positive things and people. My husband and I were able to spend February in a beach vacation rental. The month away from the cold winter was a blessing during the Covid-19 time away from family and friends. I am also grateful for an increase in my faith. Even though the Sunday Church service are too hard to navigate, I have been able to attend a weekday service at a small, local chapel, online resources, books, and phone apps.

Thank you for reading my story. I hope my experience might help someone. I will continue to remind myself that I am not in control. Trust in the Lord with all your heart; and lean not unto your own understanding (Proverbs 3: 5). Traci Lundy

MY EXPERIENCE WITH COMPLEX REGIONAL PAIN SYNDROME (CRPS)
Lindsey Beier

I had never heard of complex regional pain syndrome (CRPS) before. In 2017, I had learned of what CRPS was, and they diagnosed me with this condition.

In February 2017, I had moved into a new Flat with my Dad. We had been unpacking, moving furniture, and trying to fix some draws that had broken during the move. I remember one day, while I was wearing slipper socks, I was trying to fix some draws with my Dad. There was a plastic moving bag on the floor as I was still unpacking clothes and trying to organise everything. As I went to grab some clothes I had on my bed, I suddenly slipped and tripped over the plastic bag. I fell sideways and heard what sounded like a crack. I was not sure what had happened; it was a blur, but I just felt I could not move my leg, and I was in a lot of pain.

Afterward, after my Dad finally helped me on to the sofa in our lounge, I had said to him how bad the pain was, but I was not sure what had happened. He said to me we should just use ice to stop the swelling (you should never use ice to treat a CRPS patient, but we did not know this at the time). I remember feeling like my lower leg, and foot felt numb, but also a painful feeling whenever I tried to move, it felt like a sharp, extremely uncomfortable, no strength pain. It also felt that when I was just trying to move my lower right leg, I had a load of 10 bricks on it; it was and is still very difficult to explain.

Eventually, when the pain got worse, as we thought at the beginning, I may have had just hurt my leg, and it would heal, we went to A & E. I was told I needed a few scans and tests. I remember still feeling it was all a blur, but

I was still confused. The pain felt like it was getting worse, and the pain felt more painful than the initial injury itself.

After several days, I saw an orthopedic specialist who had reviewed my scans and tests. I was then told that I had a condition called complex regional pain syndrome (CRPS) in my right foot and leg. My Dad was in the room with me, and we both asked the orthopedic, what does that mean? It confused me and was not aware of this chronic condition.

After, I felt like I was 'couch-bound,' I found it very difficult just to stand for a few seconds, to get from one room to the next without any support. Even when I was wearing the 'big black support boot,' that the hospital gave me, I still found it difficult. I was also told to keep trying to exercise my leg and move around, though I felt I had no strength at all. There were times when my Dad if he needed to go out or to work, he would leave kitchen chairs around the flat just to help me get from one room to another, it was very painful though, and a lot of the time I remember I had to crawl. In the hospital, I would need to use a wheelchair just to get to my appointments.

By 2018, after being in and out of hospital and doctor appointments, I had started to gain some strength, but the pain was still unbearable. I was finally out of my black boot and was given extra insoles from the hospital to wear in my trainers for comfort. I was terrified of walking anywhere without any shoes on in case I would fall. I was told that for half the day to do physio exercises, and also to keep moving as much as I could, and rest when I needed to.

In late 2018, and early 2019, I remember people asking me, 'why are you not better yet? It was over a year ago that you had your injury?' I tried to explain to them I have a condition called CRPS. The number of times they would ask me, 'what is that?' Though I had already told them before what it was. I cannot even count. It was not their fault though, as it is an unknown condition. However, I felt like I was just constantly repeating myself.

I was still going to my doctor's appointments, and I was worried about the pain I was having. I started noticing the pain had spread to my right knee. I did not understand what was happening? I knew from research that CRPS can spread, but the pain in my knee was so severe that I was just not sure. After I had an MRI, which had shown it was 'all clear.' They advised me it is possible that maybe the CRPS has spread to my knee? I started wearing a bandage or tight jeggings to compress the pain. Though it still felt uncomfortable.

I contacted a UK based charity that raises awareness for CRPS and offers support to those who have this condition. The lady whom I spoke to was very nice and understanding. I remember asking her sorry, but do you know anyone personally that has CRPS because I have not met anyone that does? She told me she has CRPS herself and that some charities' volunteers have it too. I felt a relief in a way, having someone I could talk to who knows about this condition, not only that but has it herself so I could say anything without feeling judged. She told me her story; I thought it was very inspiring and helpful. I decided I wanted to do the same for others.

A specialist at a pain clinic who saw me and advised me, I should try certain pain medications. I know medications can be helpful for some people, but for others, they do not help. Everyone is different. I decided to decline on the offer of taking pain medication because of my personal experience with certain medications I have used in the past. Instead, I tried products like natural herbs, I cut caffeine out from my diet, and started drinking smoothie protein shakes to try to build up muscle, as I had muscle waste, I also started using hot pad patches whenever, I had those 'icy cold sensations' where my leg felt like it was in a bucket of ice, painful, and freezing.

Now, in 2020, I have accepted that this is a part of my life. CRPS is not who I am, but it is a part of me. I will have bad days, sometimes flare-ups. Even on days, which I consider okay, I still feel the pain. I rest when I need to, try to watch my diet, and use products and herbs, which help reduce inflammation. I still have pain; I still wear a bandage around my knee or use tight jeggings. I still have days where I feel I cannot do much, and I have days where I know I need to rest. I am still waiting to do pain management.

I now do volunteering work with a UK based charity that raises awareness for CRPS. I am hoping to get back into a career in the Performing Arts. This condition has changed my life, but I will not let it define me.

One thing I have learned is that it is okay to have days where you are feeling down, isolated, having terrible anxiety, feeling confused, and you cannot get the things you wanted to get done, done. Listen to your body and know that you are not alone. I have also learned when I am having a terrible day; I say to myself; I have had it worse before, and I have managed to get through the day, so I can now get through today. My best advice to anyone suffering from any chronic pain condition is to never give up.

IS THIS REALLY MY LIFE OR AM I DREAMING?

MY NINE-YEAR JOURNEY LIVING WITH CRPS
Kiki Sanchez

It was a beautiful August morning in 2011. I was a construction worker with the Local Union 731. I loved what I did for a living, and being a woman working alongside the men, it was a hard job, and I had a lot to prove. I always held my own and enjoyed it too. I worked for a great company. I had to be at work posted on the same block I had been at for the past two years. I had the normal 7:00 a.m., startup, which meant I had to be there by 6:45 a.m., to set up before we closed the road off. My crew was setting up for the road paving they were doing that morning. I set up the drums, and my huge "Road Closed" sign. For two years, I was dealing with the angry residents of the neighborhood because we were closing-off their road to install new sewer systems. Boy, were many of them angry. While talking to a patron of the local pharmacy that morning, a woman in a car pulled up and demanded that I open up the road to let her through the roadblock. I explained that my crew was there paving and that I could not open up the road. She got back into her car and stepped on her gas pedal. It all happened so fast, I was hit. I was not knocked over so of course me being the tough cookie that I am, I felt I was fine although, I felt this excruciating burning in my legs right under both of my knees. I still did not want to let it show. So, I acted like I was just fine. The patron I had been speaking with had called 911. An ambulance showed up right away. Of course, I knew the EMS crew as they are always allowed down my closed road because it was the major road to the hospital. I told them I was fine, and that they had nothing to check out. They saw it differently as they watched me limp to my car in pain.

At that point, the pain was so severe that I could no longer hide it. I was told to get into the ambulance and given one of those paper robes that hospitals and doctors' offices are so fond of giving to patients. Once they uncovered my legs, you could see how swollen my legs were, with the right leg being much worse. They took me to Staten Island University Hospital at once and let go with a diagnosis of bone bruising and a note giving me a few days off of work. Although I was still feeling the pain and a crazy sensitivity in my legs, all I wanted to do was go back to work. In the construction business, if you do not work, they do not pay you.

So, all I was thinking of was losing a week's pay. When I returned to work, after about forty-minutes of being on my feet, I went to speak to our safety coordinator. We decided I would file for Workman's Compensation. I went to see my orthopedic doctor soon after, and they gave me a script for physical therapy. My physical therapist began with icing down both legs. The sensitivity part of my leg pain was difficult to deal with, but with not knowing what was wrong, I dealt with it. Each time he removed the ice packs, the part of each leg that was very affected would always stay white. We know they apply ice to help treat swelling, and the area being treated should turn red from the ice packs. Since I did not have a diagnosis, my therapist was afraid and did not want me to exercise, because he was very concerned that any physical activity may cause more problems for my legs.

After a few times, I also felt that the ice may cause damage because, over time, the sensitivity to the affected area became crazy. It felt as if I had a million red ants inside my legs, and it felt as if they were chewing, gnawing, and setting fire to every area they chewed on.

So, since I was now exhibiting signs of extreme sensitivity in my legs, I would not let anybody near them. After a few months, my orthopedist

127

realized that he was not helping my situation. He referred me to a colleague that was a knee specialist. Touching or breathing on my legs was unbearable. I need you to understand something about me even though; I have a high tolerance for pain. I know that God creates us all individually. When God molded me, he gave me one gift, the ability to handle any pain that I would suffer from when getting hurt physically. I tell you this because since I handle pain well; I was consistently unsure if the doctors were grasping what I was going through.

Also, as a woman working in a male-dominated industry, showing any kind of pain means weakness. I was this tough cookie that was falling weak because of this burning pain unknown to me, and it would get worse through the years. After a few months of being treated by my orthopedic doctor's colleague, he told me he was confident that he knew what my problem was. The only problem was he could not diagnose me, and if he could diagnose me, he still could not prescribe the medication needed to treat me.

The doctor then referred me over to another colleague that was well versed in the area of complex regional pain syndrome (CRPS). At this point, I still did not know what the heck was causing this horrible burning pain in my legs. I go for my first appointment with this new doctor. While he was looking at my legs, he could see how much more swollen the right leg was.

After about a thirty-second inspection of the leg, he told me that he was pretty sure he knew what was wrong with me. Without real warning, he tells me that what he was about to do would hurt, so I started to brace myself. He took his thumb and placed it right where my right leg was most swollen, he not only touched it, but he pushed his thumb so deep into that injured area, and swear I almost kicked him.

With tears in my eyes and feeling that agonizing and excruciating pain that was burning so much, more than I have ever felt he told me I had CRPS, and handed me a pamphlet about his practice and told me to go on their website and read up on my disease, and left the room. Then his assistant walked into the room and started to explain about the medicine the doctor wanted me to take for the pain. She then said I was all set, and they would see me next month. I left the office with a prescription for Lyrica.

I do not remember how long it took after I began the Lyrica, but shortly after starting my new script, I began to hate myself and almost walked in front of an oncoming 18-wheeler. I honestly do not remember what stopped me, but the following day I was at the doctor's office in tears. I was taken off the Lyrica and given a prescription for Cymbalta. That drug was not much better.

After a short period of being on Cymbalta, each time I was at one of my son's baseball games, and it was a sunny day, I would feel like the sun was burning right through my skin and bones. I was taken off of the Cymbalta promptly and referred to my new doctor's partner in the practice that specialized in spinal cord injections.

The doctor started me on a very aggressive regimen of medications, which included the following: Exalgo (time-released) (hydromorphone) 32 mg twice a day, Oxycodone, Neurontin (a seizures medication, and it also works for nerve damage pain), Soma, muscle relaxers, and Lexapro an antidepressant. He also scheduled me for my first round of nerve block injections.

I was never pain-free, but the medications and the nerve blocks did help me. As time went on, my mom was very concerned about me and the long-term side-effects the medications could have on me. The problem I had; I was not doing the extensive research that I should have been doing on CRPS. I learned a hard lesson during one of my office visits when I questioned my doctor about the medications I was on. Well, what a mistake that was. My doctor became angered as if I was questioning who he was as a doctor. He then informed me he was no longer interested in treating me as a patient.

Being the strong-minded woman, that I am, I got my last prescriptions not fully understanding what would happen to me without my medication and nor did my doctor do the ethical thing to make sure I would still get treatment and refer me to another specialist.

When I walked into his office on that first day, I should have done more than just read about CRPS from their website. I was in so much pain at that point, and I was going through the side effects of the different medications he prescribed to me. I trusted that the doctor had it all under control. I also trusted my orthopedic doctor and his referral.

I never doubted the second opinion, but to be referred again to a third doctor even though he did not know what I was suffering from, I was just happy that each doctor could see I was in pain and that they did not dismiss me. I regret not doing a thorough search for all the information that I could get on CRPS. I trusted my doctors, and I had no reason not to trust them, right? After all, they are doctors, and my pain levels were off the charts, and they were helping me control my pain.

After all of my years of research, I have come to two conclusions: first, knowing what I know now, and my fourth doctor and his aggressive treatment of CRPS is the best way they should treat this disease in the beginning. This can also be helpful to newly diagnosed patients, within the first six to eight months after the onset of CRPS. Second, if I did not stop being treated aggressively, I could have possibly gone into remission? I am not a doctor to tell you I am positively sure that being treated aggressively would have given me a chance of going into remission? Considering my understanding of all the research that I have done along with the basic understanding of the human body and using plain old common sense, I honestly believe that my fourth doctor's treatment was the right choice. It is too late to fret about it now.

For everybody reading my story, whether you are the person who has CRPS or a family member, spouse, or loved one, please start your research right away, and do not stop because you have to learn as much as you can about this disease. There will always be newer treatments and medications, and so many people who claim to be experts within the medical community. Still, many doctors and nurses do not know enough about this disease that has been around since the 18th century.

Most often, the patient has to be his or her advocate and has to open the eyes of many people within a medical staff, whether at the emergency rooms or within a new doctor's office. It is crucial to most CRPS cases that the diagnosed patient arm themselves with all the knowledge possible. So many procedures can end up harming a CRPS patient, especially if the attending physician believes that the pain the patient is describing "is all in the patient's head." Sadly, this is all too often the case. So please, do the research. Kommentar [WD1]: Back to my journey now.

I am on my last few weeks of medications. I was not ready to deal with the consequence of just going off my medications. What did I know about prescription medications? I knew nothing of what I was about to go through. A few days after I stopped taking my medications, I felt flu-like symptoms. A few days later, I thought I could be hospitalized. I was so sick and could not seem to sleep.

This was a painful six months. By the time my body could function without the medications, the CRPS came back and seemed to come back with a vengeance, as if during the detox, it was being held captive. I was not only flooded with pain, but emotionally I was not sure if I could handle the agony CRPS was inflicting on my body. While my family slept, I would be awake in tears. Not once did I ever let one person know what I was going through emotionally. When my kids were in school, it became harder and harder to clean my house or cook a meal. I love being in the kitchen. Now, instead of looking forward to cooking, and I had to get excited about what food we would order. Taking my dogs out for a walk also became a challenge.

Over time, I became much more knowledgeable about this disease, and with everything; I read and the more I learned, I swore that I could never possibly get any worse like the stories I was reading online. As time passed, and each time the pain got worse or spread, I had to admit to myself that I was not the special person who would or could spontaneously go into remission. I knew then that things could only get worse. So, I prayed for the best and prepared for the worst. Still, I showed no one that I was having some concerns about how the disease was eating me from the inside out. So now after that crazy detox, I knew I needed to find a doctor ASAP, but a doctor who had some knowledge about CRPS.

After calling many doctor offices and being told from the start that their doctors will not prescribe me any medications, I finally found a new pain management doctor, Doctor NS. I was immediately placed back on some of my medications, and this time before my new doctor handed me all of my scripts, he asked me what I wanted to do. He gave me options for my treatment. He made me feel that I needed to be involved in the decision-making of my treatment.

I have been with him for almost six years now. He asked me to try a spinal cord stimulator (SCS) in the beginning too. When the leads moved during the trial period, it gave my legs even more pain. I also read up on a few CRPS patients who had difficulties with the SCS and the surgeries, leaving them in more pain. By then, the stimulator was not the way to go.

After a few months of being Doctor S., patient, I was in a car accident in January 2015. A box truck hit my car then forced into the concrete jersey barrier. In an instant, my pain shot to new higher levels that I had never felt before. I was at Doctor S's., office immediately. I had MRI's done because my back and legs were in so much pain. I was in terrible shape. Not only was my disease getting worse, but now I was suffering neck and back pain. How much more could I possibly take??

I now had days that were so intense, more than not. A depression that I never saw coming because I feel like I am so strong, it was a depression-like one I have never felt. I spent most of my alone time in tears. I never thought I could get any worse. I was so determined to fight. Boy, have I fought I tried to walk and exercise, and it still got worse! The exercising and walking would force me into bed for days from the constant pain, burning pain, and sensitivity.

To help my neck and back pain they referred me to a chiropractor. It is hard to manipulate my back because of the aftershock of pain that I get in my spine. Working on my neck is all he could do, and trust me, I had my days when I could not see him at all. My chiropractor learned my moods, whether I was in extreme physical pain or not. He could see when I wanted to breakdown and just cry. He referred me over to a therapist, by the name of Doctor AW., because he felt I needed to talk about how this has affected my life. I never dealt with my emotional pain. Just putting this story together brought out so many emotions, and I have not even told you about how much worse I have gotten.

Just a slight brush up against my legs from my dog sends me into a downward spiral. Banging my hand on the door frame can send shooting pain from that hand through the entire arm. I have to be careful with anything that I do once I am out of bed. My body has become so fragile, and there are still CRPS patients who suffer worse than I do. I thank God, every day that I have Doctor AW., to talk to. She comes to my home if I cannot make it to her. Driving has become difficult.

I taught myself how to drive with my left leg and have even used cruise control on the highways. Now, my oldest son drives me around.

Things have been hard to accept. I hate asking for help. I always saw it as a sign of weakness. Some days, I hate myself for needing so much help. About six months after my last car accident, I began having terrible sinus trouble. My sinuses were draining straight into my throat, covering my airways. For two-years, no doctor took me seriously regarding my problem. I found an ENT specialist, and a year after trying to use nasal sprays to control the problem to no avail, he sent me for a sonogram of my facial cavity. One day later, my doctor was on the phone telling me how serious the problem was. I had a deviated septum, and I needed surgery, and he also said that most doctors help patients with a nasal spray, so surgery was rare if not avoided for this issue.

We also talked about how this surgery could make my CRPS spread to my face. I needed this surgery, or my breathing would never be normal again. So, I had the surgery, and at first, I was just fine. After almost two weeks later, I began to feel this fire in my face that even causes my gums and teeth to hurt. Some days, I wake up, and my face has the red patches that burn me and render me useless for the day.

Now, after some more time, I was just progressing at a faster rate. Since my last car accident, my body just continues to get exceptionally worse. When I get stressed out, I get these weird red patches on my legs that almost look like a rash that feels like they are burning me from the inside out. They affect both of my arms too. My left is worse than my right, but both burn like hell. I cannot be on my feet too much, or my legs and ankles swell up something fierce. I also had a terrible experience a few years ago.

One night, I was lying in bed, and I felt hot. So hot that it felt as I was melting from inside the core of my body. Then, a few seconds later, I felt so cold. It was like I was freezing from inside the core of my body. This issue went back and forth for over an hour. My mom had me rushed to the hospital. I felt as I was going to die.

By the time we made it to the hospital, I was already feeling better. They wanted to keep me overnight to monitor my body temperature. The attending doctor was afraid that my CRPS was the cause. I just wanted to go home. Since that day, my core body temperature seems to always be on the hotter side. At 44-years of age, if I feel well enough, I try to go food shopping but have to ride in the scooters that the stores provide, or it will take me near three hours to complete my shopping. My big toenails look so damn bad too.

Once my legs got worse, the nails on my big toes became cracked and broke. I would get these horrible ingrown nails on each toe. It is hard to wear certain types of shoes too. I found wearing Crocs are the most comfortable, no more high heels or boots. I used to get my nails done until my hands started showing symptoms of CRPS. Sometimes, I cannot sign my name with my left hand when I am having a flare-up. I have had days when my husband has to carry me to and from the bathroom. How sad is that? I need more help than I ask for cleaning the house because it has become too difficult for me. If my kids and my husband did not do my chores, my house would never be clean. My pride is very strong. It kills me I can no longer do the things I used to do before I developed CRPS.

I understand that when you take the vow of marriage; it is in sickness and in health. I have read about so many marriages that end because the healthy partner could not deal with their other half being sick. My husband is the most wonderful man in the world. How amazing it is that he supports me and is always by my side through these years since my diagnosis. I love him so much.

When I take a shower, I get the worse pain ever. The water feels like shards of glass going through my skin. My husband put a seat in the shower for me, and he changed the showerhead, making it easier for me to shower without the water beating on my body. He is there to help me get dressed.

My kids help by doing chores like the laundry and making sure there are no dishes in the sink. They even clean their bathroom. Full family support is so important. Even my mom spends weekends with me to cook a few meals for the week for my family. She cleans and helps with everything.

She takes off from work to drive and accompany me to my doctor's appointments for moral support. I hate having to baby my body and letting my family clean for me now, but I have no choice. I cannot do all these things anymore.

On most days, I feel like a prisoner in my body and my house. I hate to go out because people can be so barbaric. I move so slowly that I irritate people, and they always show their annoyance. That makes me feel not only angry but hurts me. I am now partially disabled. I still cannot wrap my head around it! To be honest, the hardest part has been accepting my limitations. I cry so much that I am surprised that I still have tears to shed. Sometimes I swear that the pain in my heart burns more than my body during a flare-up. I hate the days I wake up feeling good, and once I move around my calves burn, and it starts, a nasty flare-up, that forces me back to bed. I refuse to give up!

With support from my family, amazing doctors, and my trust in God, I am learning to accept this disease and my limitations. Little by little, I am also learning to accept help from others. I hope my story shows that living with CRPS; is not the end of the world. I know that there are days that seem so dark and hard to snap out of it. If you find yourself in that terrible place, please try to reach out to a therapist, family member, or a trusted friend, and release all that emotional stress that you are holding deep down inside.

We have to educate doctors about CRPS; because of a few patients, and this leads to more research by these doctors. If you are not happy with your doctor, as hard as it is, do your research and find yourself another doctor. Please, NEVER, EVER, give up because you ARE important!

MY THORN AND MY FIGHT
Donna L. Artis

It all began with me telling my husband of 13-years that the wind from the fan was hurting me. He had a normal reaction of what? He did not understand it and laughed. I was still recovering from yet-another attempt to fix my left foot because of a failed bunionectomy. This surgery was my third in less than two years. I never imagined how this event would forever change my life and the many adjustments I would need. I would have so many emotions hit me and hit hard that it became very difficult and frustrating to explain exactly what my diagnosis was to my friends and family. First, I would have to learn what I had. They diagnosed with complex regional pain syndrome (CRPS), or also known as reflex sympathetic dystrophy (RSD).

Amazing how four letters would forever change who I had been for 34-years. It all began with a much-needed bunionectomy and a cyst removal on my left foot. I had already had one done on my right foot and had no issues. This foot would need a steel plate and more screws to help keep my foot aligned and healed. This issue was in 2014 when the screw became loose and started pushing through the top of my foot. I had another x-ray that showed the screw was too long and would be removed and replaced with a shorter screw, and there was another cyst on the bottom of my foot, needed to be removed. This surgery was in April 2015. When I had this surgery, I was told that it would take care of the problems. WRONG!!! I went back to my podiatrist and told him, six months later, that the pain was still there, and I was not getting better. After more x-rays, the podiatrist said that the metal had not mended and my foot bones were not healing. He said I needed another surgery, one that would replace all the metal and screws in my foot with new and shorter materials. They also had to take a bone graft and have it screwed to my foot and the metal because my bones needed more to heal closed. For this surgery, I received a bone growth stimulator that I had to use it every day, twice daily for 30-minutes. I did this for about a month then I was told to stop. The recovery time now was up to 12-weeks. I became so accustomed to the calf-length brace that for the next year I only wore it and a right-side regular shoe. It's sad! Knowing now what I did not know then, I would have reconsidered.

Fast forward to December 2015–April 2016 and the news. I had to have another surgery because again, one screw was coming out and poking me through the skin, making shoes impossible to wear. I switched foot doctors and was told that the length of the screw could have been why my cyst kept coming back and why I had the sensitivity to my shoes and socks. Well, the night before my follow-up appointment, and after the surgery finalizations, the air from the fan hurt me.

It was so weird and at first; I laughed because I thought it was so silly. It was not! I posted my situation on Facebook, and instantaneously I was told my symptoms sounded like CRPS. Huh? It shocked me when I looked up the symptoms and the diagnosis of this disease. I had all the symptoms discussed. I had non-stop pain, my foot would be colder or hotter than the rest of my body, and I had severe swelling; I also had had multiple surgeries in the same area in a brief amount of time that caused irreversible nerve damage. Also, I have a sensitivity to the wind and sound. Everything fit! I waited until I had my appointment a few days later, and I brought it up to my podiatrist. He said yes; he determined all the symptoms fit, and that is what he would tell me the diagnosis was.

What made me laugh is after he tells me having more surgeries or traumatic injuries can spread CRPS. I have to have another surgery! For real? I could not believe the road I was going to taking.

I had worked for my company who was a contractor for mortgage companies, banks, insurance, and homeowner claims. I loved my job; loved the details and ability to multitask. Well, between starting physical therapy and having what I would learn were flares, and I was out of work on FMLA. I quickly learned physical therapy did NOT work for helping my pain. I would be in a flare for a few days after a session, so I stopped. I became scared of even having my blood taken because it can be spread that easy. Then the other symptoms started: brain fog, vertigo, sensitivity to sound, sensitivity to touch and vibration, the use of a cane to keep me stable, scooters for outings and store shopping, CHRONIC FATIGUE SYNDROME, and more. They were all embarrassing to me because I was still "young." I would be in mid-conversation with someone, and immediately my mind would go blank. I could blame the medicine they had me try as well as the CRPS.

When the doctor first diagnosed with CRPS, he placed me on Gabapentin and Tramadol for pain. Well, neither of those helped, and, for a year I was taking the Gabapentin, I gained 80-pounds! It was not because of inactivity or just eating, but because it is a side effect of this nerve medicine. Taking Tramadol did nothing for the pain, but there are many other choices. CRPS is a disease, a rare one at that. I have an invisible disease, but I also had to learn how to become my own best advocate. Trying to find a doctor who knew about CRPS was next to impossible.

I had to explain the disease and bring up treatment options to my doctors and continuously document my skin discoloration, swelling, lifestyle, and anything that changed my daily life.

I joined many support groups online and realized, that this may be a rare disease, but the number of people who had this was probably like me who at first never got an official diagnosis. The symptoms are very similar to fibromyalgia, which is a disease almost everyone knew about. When I found out this disease has been around since the Civil War, and I was amazed there has been very little done research-wise, to find a cure. It is infuriating! It is infuriating! There is no 100% definitive test. Instead, the test for CRPS is based on the Budapest criteria. It is a checklist of symptoms, and depending on how many you say yes to, that gives the medical professional a basis to back up the diagnosis. I have a very understanding family doctor who did all she could to help me, but I needed more help than what she could just offer me. They referred me to a pain management doctor who has been a godsend. They gave me a permanent disability placard. A funny side note; I had been getting a six-month temporary placard for a year when my pain management doctor finally wrote me a script for a permanent one. When I went into the license bureau with my script, the teller said, it is about time they give you a permanent one! I said really? I could not help laughing. It was also at the time I ran out of FMLA time at my job. So, I had to decide if I should quit and apply somewhere else or file for disability.

I prayed to find a job that could be flexible with my flares or brain fog episodes and doctor appointments. Yeah, it did not happen.

In September, my husband and I made a decision that I should apply for SSD. I was nervous because I know how hard it is for someone to get approved with a well-known issue, let alone a rare and unknown disease. The waiting for a decision was so hard, along with the struggles of having no income and the lack of meaning in life. Depression is just as common with chronic pain as brain fog. Well, I finally got my decision on November

15, 2017, and they approved my disability! I was shocked. As we know, patients suffering from CRPS do not get better, only worse, and after being examined by a psychologist from Social Security, I passed. I say failed but passed per their disability standards. It was bittersweet. Here, I was 35-years-old and legally disabled. IT SUCKED!!

They referred me to a pain management doctor who has been a godsend. In February 2018, I began receiving Ketamine infusions and nerve blocks. None of the prescribed medication would help, and my pain was a constant 7-10 on the pain scale. It is amazing what our bodies do to adjust to living in a constant state of pain. My first infusion was strange. Ketamine is a known horse tranquilizer but also known on the streets as Special K. I did not understand they had used it for successful treatment, NOT a cure, for CRPS patients, and to help with the symptoms. They did the nerve block in my lower back to go down to my main affected limb. It is a treatment that takes time to build up in your system before you can notice any changes. After about three months of getting these treatments once a month in the hospital, I could finally start feeling a change. Now, my pain levels were between three and seven, instead of a constant minimum of seven. I also was using marijuana on the side to help with pain and sleeplessness that goes along with having chronic pain. Things were better, but I knew there were other treatment options.

In January 2019, my doctor contacted me to be a part of a medical study involving Neridronate Acid. Doctors in Italy have been doing this treatment for about 10-years now, and it has shown a small success rate of sending CRPS into remission. I had to go through medical testing and tons of blood work. My doctor informed me that my Vitamin-D level was at 11 when the normal range should be between 30-60. It was low, so I had to take a high dose of Vitamin-D, and get retested every two weeks to check my levels because I needed mine to be at 30 before, they would allow me to be in the study.

Well, I finally hit 30 at the end of February, so they cleared me to take part in the study. The downside was that I had to stop my Ketamine infusion treatments and the nerve blocks for the duration of the trial study. OUCH! The trial included four infusions of either a placebo or a dose of Neridronate Acid. I had to keep a daily journal of my pain, and the constant blood draws. I had to have two, four-hour infusions a week for two weeks. It may not sound like a lot, but when you constantly get needles put in your arms for the I.V. and another needle for blood work, it becomes overwhelming.

Things were improving, and I was looking forward to the last set of infusions because they were guaranteed to use Neridronate Acid. Then, I received a phone call in June that the medical company had canceled the research study because they did not see a high enough number of people getting relief. I cannot even describe my disappointment, but I immediately called my pain management doctor, and he said I could begin the Ketamine infusions again.

Slowly but surely, my body buildup, and the relief became more constant. I am always not in pain, but if my level is between two and four. That is an exceptional day! Now I take Kratom and use marijuana to help with my symptoms and pain. My pain management doctor is all for anything natural to help my pain. He also placed me on a low dose of Naltrexone, which has made an enormous difference.

I have become a very active warrior in the CRPS community for spreading awareness and knowledge of this disease for others. I have received Ohio's Proclamation for November as being "CRPS Awareness Month."

My family and friends have become more educated, and they help me spread awareness. This disease has caused me to lose many friends due to suicide because they cannot take the pain, depression, frustration, or loneliness of this beast. Every few months I seem to lose a friend because they just cannot take it anymore. This disease starts in one limb but quickly can spread. I get flares in my hands and face as well; I have had to leave certain events and even church because the sounds become too hurtful. I still have days of depression, but I also have my faith to get me through it. I know God has a plan for me, and I just need to submit and follow the path he has for me and CRPS.

I am blessed to have an understanding and empathetic husband who has helped spread awareness in the EMT field and other friends in the hospitals.

I refuse to let this disease beat me. I fight for support and awareness and I will never stop. There may be no cure for CRPS, but I pray I can be a part of a study that is working on a cure for future generations.

I would like to share one of my favorite biblical quotes.

The Thorn in the Flesh

And lest I should be exalted above measure by the abundance of the revelations, a thorn in the flesh was given to me, a messenger of Satan to buffet me, lest I be exalted above measure. Concerning this thing, I pleaded with the Lord three times that it might depart from me. And He said to me, "My grace is sufficient for you, for My strength is made perfect in weakness." Therefore, most gladly I will rather boast in my infirmities, that the power of Christ may rest upon me. Therefore, I take pleasure in infirmities, in reproaches, for Christ's sake. FOR WHEN I AM WEAK, THEN I AM STRONG! – (2 Corinthians 12:7-10 New King James Version)

A CRPS PATIENT'S STORY
P.S.

My complex regional pain syndrome (CRPS) story started in August 2013, after I had surgery on my left leg, to remove a benign tumor that was near the sciatic nerve at the top of my hamstring. An orthopedic surgeon, Doctor M.J., performed the surgery at the Cleveland Clinic (he died from ALS). What may have caused the tumor in the first place was falling on black ice in 1999. What I learned is that a percussive injury may cause swelling and that will dissipate after healing. What may also occur is the development of a benign tumor, which may have been the case for me. I had been dealing with sciatic nerve pain for years before the finding of the tumor with many attempts at treatment, not knowing that there was a tumor involved.

About nine months after my surgery, the doctor diagnosed me with CRPS. After the nerves grew back, the pain never went away. I knew that this was not normal as I had previous surgeries without having such a reaction.

Doctor K.G. was the first pain management doctor that I saw. He was not a compassionate nor helpful doctor. His solution to my pain was to provide me with drugs, which all of them had adverse and intolerable side-effects. He eventually told me (rather rudely) that he could no longer see me as a patient as he did not know what to do with me. I saw him from the winter of 2013 to the spring of 2014. I eventually went to see someone new (Doctor M.N.).

Doctor M.N., was leading a study for the DRG stimulator. He saw my situation, and he suggested I try a spinal cord stimulator (SCS). I ended up in the control group, and they gave me a Medtronic SCS (vs. what I came to learn was the DRG stimulator). Since Doctor M.N.; was leading the

145

study, it was a conflict of interest for him to continue seeing me. He decided to refer me to see Doctor S. S., who did my surgeries and my treatments from then on. I had immediate relief from the test stimulator and had the permanent device implanted in August 2014, which only helped for about a year.

I now see that I was helping Doctor M.N., with his study, but it was also a chance for me to get some relief.

Over the years, I have had many surgeries for other issues before CRPS, but they are unrelated. Below is a list of surgeries I have had related only to my CRPS:

- Spinal cord stimulator – A regular Medtronic as part of the Accurate study. The trial was done first, which brought tremendous relief. The permanent SCS was implanted in August of 2014.

- Hydro-dissection surgery was done to try to separate the scar tissue from the nerve. It succeeded in doing that, but it increased the pain instead of helping.

- Surgery in September of 2019 was done to remove the old SCS referenced above. It only helped for about a year when my brain got used to it and no longer provided any benefit.

- DRG stimulator trial was done in October of 2019. I received limited benefit in my foot, but it brought enough relief to do the permanent device, which was done in December 2019.

I have been back to the doctor five times to have the DRG stimulator adjusted as it has not been helping. I have been on hold due to the Covid-19 situation.

Over the years, I have tried every medication imaginable, all with negative side-effects. One of the worst was Gralise (Gabapentin). This medication caused a change in my personality. It made me angry and caused me to do and say inappropriate things, and that's not me. My husband (God-bless him) only thought it was the pain, and not realizing it was the medication, which took a few months to take this effect, and a few months to taper off. That time in my life is a blur in my mind and disturbing to recollect. The only medications I take are Vicodin 5-325 mg; I am only allowed two pills total per day and Gabapentin 900 mg per day (all I can tolerate).

In December 2016, I had tried a Ketamine treatment with a new doctor. The reason for going somewhere else was because my regular doctor had a 14-month waiting list for the Ketamine treatment. This experience was one of the worst treatments of my life. I could not move the entire time and had horrible hallucinations of death. This event was awful. I had no relief at all. The doctor convinced me to try a second day of treatment, which was a mistake. It was a total failure!

In August 2017, I had a procedure called hydro-dissection to separate the scar tissue from the sciatic nerve. An orthopedic doctor did this surgery, not my regular pain management doctor. We considered the procedure a success as it separated the scar tissue from the nerve. Unfortunately, this surgery made the pain worse instead of better.

I have tried physical therapy over the years without success, included water-therapy. I am to the point in which being in the water at all, causes me increased pain. I cannot go into a hot tub, pool, or bathtub at all.

The water pressure is intolerable. Part of physical therapy also included dry needling. One of the sessions caused a terrible hematoma with blood pooling under the skin, and eruption that caused a tremendous amount of discomfort and pain.

Massage therapy helps. Unfortunately, that is an out-of-pocket payment and is expensive. It took some time to find a good therapist, and she makes home visits. I have her visit me when I can. She cannot touch my affected leg anymore, but she helps with the hip area where I have pain because of degenerative disc disease.

In September 2019, I had the Medtronic SCS removed. I also had an MRI done while I could check the status of my spine and the former location of the tumor that started this mess. I was trying to obtain the DRG stimulator for over two years, but insurance (United Healthcare) rejected it as experimental and unproven. I engaged a lawyer but to no avail. I have been on disability since July 2017 and waited until I was eligible for Medicare. That got me approval right away.

I had a DRG stimulator trial in October 2019. During the first few days of using the trial stimulator, it did not provide me with any relief. I met with the representative from Medtronic, and he made some adjustments, and I had some relief in the foot, enough to warrant the full device. The doctor installed the permanent stimulator in December 2019. Unfortunately, they could not place the lead at the S-1 level, which is where I needed it the most. Since then, I have been back several times to change the stimulator programs with no relief. It was my last resort. I am on my last four programs, and I am testing them out. Setting the stimulator too high causes me more pain. So far, it is not helping me.

I did everything I could to continue working, but this was no longer possible. My employer laid me off in January 2017, and I applied for disability soon after, and they approved me in less than three months. That was a wake-up call for me as it showed that the CRPS had messed up (less than seven percent get approved on their first try in my area).

Fortunately, my husband has been supportive and fantastic throughout. We moved last year to a new home more conducive to my condition. I am not addicted to any medications, but I do rely on Vicodin for some relief. I am not homeless, and I am not suicidal. I get depressed, but not tremendously so, as I am a pretty positive person.

Thank you for reading my story.

LIFE'S BIRTHDAY GIFT
Lisa Deere

Some say that life is not always fair nor does it pick who receives favors or despair, but in reality, the saying "Bad things happen to good people," reflects on how life's justification or attempt of easing those who have received more than their share of misfortune events. These are events that have made their life's journey in a series of constant illnesses, problems getting disability, missing out on enjoying their children as they grow up, children missing a parent because of illness, failed marriages and understanding the changes, and challenges that life has left us to struggle and to comprehend.

Unfortunately, the accuracy of those six simple words when put in order becomes a way for people to justify a lack of understanding of what people who have more than a life's share of unexplainable misfortune events. I am living proof of the accuracy of those six words. I have complex regional pain syndrome (CRPS), and my journey with this disease is one that I share, hoping to help anyone who is looking for answers. Please know you are not alone and take comfort from the fact that you are a warrior who can choose how you approach this battle.

My battle began in September 2016. I guessed the fact I beat Endometrial cancer at age 27 would be the worst medical condition life could and would put me through. I mean, if you have been through cancer of any type you understand what I am referring to. Going through chemotherapy, radiation, new medications (reactions to which some of them put you in the hospital), nausea, surgery, the diagnostic test, and repetitive tests, and scans help guide doctors on how your body is handling the stress in which it is going through. The only thing you want is to live and enjoy remission.

That golden opportunity in which you hope and pray for that your cancer stays away. I consider myself blessed as my cancer did not return. Seventeen years later, something started in my left foot that caused me a lot of pain that I did not understand could happen. I recognized there was something wrong, and I needed my feet healthy, so I could continue dancing and teaching fitness. Never did I imagine the journey that I was about to embark on. I believe no one saw what the future held for me, and to say as time and doctors went by, being scared for my life was an understatement. I knew my pain was moving in and up my body.

I started my medical treatment with my PCP, who swore my purple, swollen, painful foot was because of my heart and wasted nine months of my time running and re-running every heart test with the same result, NO CARDIAC PROBLEMS. Since I was a certified group fitness instructor, I worked out religiously; I eat healthy, and grew up dancing since the age of two and was a competitive soccer player until the season before CRPS took over my foot. I mean things did not add up, and I was quick to see doctors who did not have a clue, so I spent the next several months watching the pain, and swelling spread to my other foot and worked its way up my leg.

On March 8, 2019 (my birthday) after being in two hospitals in ICU because my face swelled to epic proportions, and they diagnosed me with lupus, and they sent me to see a Rheumatologist. The doctor missed the CRPS, but he sent me to a pain management group, and on my birthday, they gave me an appointment. The first doctor came in and asked me what I was being seen for? I explained I was there for my back because that is where the CRPS was taking its toll on me, or that is what I thought. The next few minutes changed my world. She said your back is secondary to your feet problem, and she left the room and came back in with her three partners and I heard it…. CRPS. I was like, huh? What is that?

They did not have any answers except for me to find a therapist, a support group and we will try to keep you out of pain. Well, happy birthday to me! The one doctor looked at several of my blood work tests I had done, and she stated, just as I should understand, that I was deficient in Vitamin-D in all of them. I did not feel like celebrating at all, especially when I read about this illness and try to make sense of it all. Unfortunately, doctors did not have the answers or wanted to look for answers, or even see me as a patient when I explained my symptoms, but I was finally diagnosed, and it was time to get help to make the pieces fit.

Now with the knowledge in hand, it was time to get a specialist and doctors to help me. Boy, was I in for the search of a lifetime giving my illness a name made me unbelievable and crazy because CRPS was like the illness that fell through the medical communities' fingers, and it was breaking me down; and in 2019 was my most defying year to establish what I was made of, and I finally realized that I was not alone.

If you suffer from CRPS, I am sure you have many stories to share concerning the complete roller coaster ride you experienced when trying to find an experienced, knowledgeable, compassionate, and respectful doctor to help us believe in us and understand us and our many needs. I have seen 34 doctors and been through three major hospitals. I have traveled from Florida to Houston and being from Dallas one would believe someone would have the answers. But they did not, or they could not treat me, or would not treat me. They place me in a psych ward at a hospital and immediately discharged the next day. It has been the loneliest time in my life, and I have missed so many things in my boy's life, and it put a strain on my recent marriage. After a year of chaos and having this disease consume me, my birthday of 2020, they scheduled to give me some pain relief. I would receive Ketamine infusions. I am not making this as a general statement but as a personal one. The Ketamine treatment worked for me, and for the first time in years, my pain was slowly going away with each treatment.

I found the most amazing PCP, Doctor F. He did not understand what CRPS was, but he was a compassionate and caring man who could say I needed help. Help and hope are what I received as he has tried to understand, read, and study with the best of his ability to help me with my crazy symptoms. He provided help in arranging my tests and procedures to prepare me for my infusions. I am very thankful to him. Because the Ketamine worked after several infusions, I am pain-free from CRPS pain, but the pain remains in some spots because CRPS will leave damage that cannot be reversed. When you suffer from CRPS, it forever changes you. I know that it is still here, just trying to push my nervous system around, and get its hold back on my body.

I can honestly say that I never in a million years thought dancing would become a part of my past. A past life that I have fought so hard to accept because of my CRPS is forever changed, and I have to acknowledge that life is something we must not take for granted. I am not mad, nor do I blame my higher power for any of this.

We now come back to those six words that I started my story with, "BAD THINGS HAPPEN TO GOOD PEOPLE." I feel that some of us may have received a bigger dose of these bad things. Over time, living in pain and suffering from CRPS, we see the bigger picture. I feel each of us has a purpose and a story to tell to help others. Remember, you are a warrior just as I am, and I refuse to go down without putting up a fight because I was not born to give up.

There is a solution out there to what plagues us. Never lose hope, and victory is possible. One day, one hour, one minute at a time, if that is what we must do to make it, and we must make it because we are warriors with a story to tell. God Bless.